HEALTHY GUT
Happy You

by Jeniffer Alburquerque, NTP

Creator of blog and recipe app Naked Flavors

Legal Notice and Disclaimer

This book is intended for educational and general information purposes only, and not as personal medical advice, medical opinion, diagnosis, or treatment. The publisher and author of this cookbook are not responsible in any manner whatsoever for any adverse effects arising directly or indirectly as a result of the information provided in this book.

Content

Cooking is more than just mixing ingredients and coming up with savory dishes. It is a way to feed your body, mind, and soul. Food unites people and when passion is one of the ingredients, it becomes a way to create memories and connect with the ones we love.

This is why I want to dedicate these next few pages to my friends and family, whom I like to call my human angels, to thank them for letting me use them as guinea pigs for the recipes in this book.

To all of you: thank you from the bottom of my heart for supporting me and motivating me to write this book. I sincerely love you all and I feel truly blessed to have you in my life. Thank you for being part of this adventure!

Acknowledgements

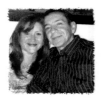

Ma' and Pa': For supporting and respecting my decisions. You were hesitant about me giving nature a chance to cure my condition, but you backed me up. Thank you for loving me so much, for being my backbone, and for letting me know you love me unconditionally.

Little bro: Thank you for being one of the main taste-testers, for always appreciating my cooking and not letting any food go to waste! I love you to pieces!

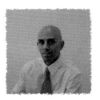

Shantih Coro: Without your guidance and patience, I wouldn't be where I am today. Thank you so much for your personalized treatment, for constantly supporting me and for always being sincere with your advice. Thank you for opening my eyes to a new and better reality. I will always be thankful that you helped me turn my health around. I have learned so much because of you, and while there's always more to learn, I feel confident sharing my knowledge and experience with others.

Alie: The universe works in inexplicable ways when you allow things to flow. Life always has your back when you are following your passion; the resources and people always show up in your path when you need them the most. This is why I am convinced that meeting you, my editor and friend, was a miracle. You became part of this writing adventure at the perfect time and unexpectedly. Alie, you have been an essential part in making this book a wonderful reality. I will forever be thankful for all your support and encouragement.

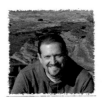

Allan: From the bottom of my heart I want to say "thank you! thank you! thank you!" You are an amazing person and I am so lucky to have you as a friend. Your support and motivation mean so much to me. Thank you for feeding into my crazy ideas, for your suggestions and for sincerely sharing my happiness throughout this writing adventure. You are one of a kind, my friend!

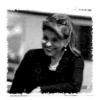

Vivian: I am so lucky our paths crossed at yoga class. Thank you so much for welcoming me to your house with open arms and for allowing me to play in your beautiful kitchen. I always felt inspired when we cooked together. Your words of encouragement and advice meant so much to me, especially because they were coming from such a wonderful and sophisticated woman.

Myrna: I love your adventurous soul! But what I love the most is having your friendship. Thank you so much for supporting my projects, for motivating me and for pushing me to be a risk-taker. You are worth more than words can express.

Jonathan: Wow! Where should I start? You appeared in my life when I least expected and took me on this magical adventure. In this short period of time, you have shown me how much you love me. Thank you for all that you do, for your support and for believing in me and in my dreams. Every day I give thanks to the universe for allowing me to share my days with such an amazing man like you. I love you with all my heart!

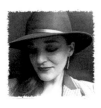

Cindy: es.tee.lo rocks! Thank you so much for styling me for the cover of Naked Flavors and for making the process of trying on thousand clothes a fun experience. Love your fun and stylish soul!

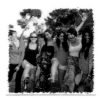 **Friends**: aka taste-testers, guinea-pigs. Thank you guys for being so supportive and encouraging, and for adding excitement to my cooking and writing experience. I love every single one of you!

Before we start...

When my health hit rock bottom, I had two options: to accept my condition and learn to live with it or to take a chance and try a method that seemed like a shot in the dark. I took a risk and decided for the second option and I made a promise to myself that if I ever healed my condition, I would do my best to inspire as many people as possible to learn to love themselves and to help them understand what a great blessing it is to be healthy. The main purpose of this book is to help whoever is looking for alternatives to recover, maintain or improve their health, and to inspire them to make the right changes to truly enjoy life to its fullest.

From the bottom of my heart I want to say thank you for choosing this book, for taking the time to read these pages and for allowing me to share my experience.

Wish you all health, love, peace and happiness,

Jen

My story

When I was 18, I began to suffer from chronic acne. I thought it was normal to have acne as a teenager, assuming it was due to hormones, and thought I would outgrow it. I tried a variety of prescription topical and oral medications, none of which permanently healed my skin.

After many trials with acne medications, I was prescribed birth control pills to help correct my hormones, and therefore clear my skin—they worked like a charm. It was simple to just pop a pill every morning and voila! No more acne!

Four years passed, during which I didn't worry about my skin at all, as I only experienced occasional small breakouts. All of the sudden, though, I began experiencing digestive problems, lack of energy, weight loss, and had trouble sleeping. Every night I would wake around 3:00 am, unable to fall back asleep. Needless to say, getting out of bed in the morning was a struggle. My acne came back with a vengeance and I felt lousy. I wasn't supposed to feel this way at such a young age.

I lost my self-confidence and self-esteem. I stopped socializing and was depressed all the time. I didn't feel like going to school or work. My grades and work performance began to fail. I couldn't stand the way I looked anymore or the path my life was taking. This person wasn't me. I felt as though I was trapped in a body that wasn't mine. Desperately seeking to find a solution, I began to scour the internet and noticed that several acne sufferers healed their conditions through diet.

Back then, my diet was not a priority. Sometimes I would get so caught up with work and school that I would forget to eat. Many days I survived on energy drinks and junk food, which further disrupted my hormones and mood, and made me even more fatigued.

I realized that my condition had become more serious than just acne. Acne was simply the first symptom of something more serious going on in my body. I was at my wit's end and ready to explore a different path in search of a cure for everything that was ailing me. I couldn't continue doing the same thing over and over again expecting different results because by definition, that is insanity!

At this point I had only two options: continue the insanity by repeating the same cycle or give nature a chance to heal me. I started my search for a holistic professional who could help me. Little did I know, the first call I made would be the start of a life-changing journey. Shantih Coro, a functional medicine practitioner in Florida, opened my eyes to the wonderful reality that my acne was only a symptom of something greater happening in my body and that there was no need to be dependent on medicine to cure it. He taught me to treat my body right and that food and lifestyle directly impact health and emotions.

During the first phase of the program, I had my doubts that nature had the power to heal, but was dedicated to giving this path a chance, as I had run out of options.

I am not going to lie: the process was not as simple as just taking a pill and watching my ailments magically disappear. It required a lot of will power and a real desire to change and improve my life. It was a cycle of ups and downs, but since the moment I began reducing my sugar intake, consuming quality foods, and consciously taking care of my emotions, my body started to heal itself. My digestion improved tremendously. I was more energetic and it was easier to wake up. I no longer needed to set three alarms to ensure I got out of bed. Best of all, my skin began to heal. I felt renewed from the inside out and there was no way I was ever turning back.

As my health began shifting in the right direction, I became passionate about the connection between the food we consume and our health. I was so impressed by how much energy I had and I started loving my body again. I didn't see it as a prison anymore; instead, it became my greatest treasure. I became more spontaneous and began recovering the social and outgoing Jen I had always been.

Now every morning that I wake up, I can touch my face and smile because those bumps have finally disappeared. Life is better, simpler and more exciting. As the changes continued, I implemented more exercise into my daily routine. I do believe that internal and external health go hand in hand. I practice yoga because it involves more than flexibility and stretching exercises. Yoga is a way of bringing peace and balance to your body and mind through mindful movement with controlled breathing. I encourage you to add movement to your life.

I have changed not only from the outside, but also from the inside. I am conscious to always continue learning. I am still discovering how wonderful and powerful our bodies and minds are. Our bodies are so complex that it takes a lifetime to understand each of its parts, but don't worry, you don't need to become a doctor or a nutritionist in order to be healthy; you simply have to start making your own life and health a priority.

My purpose with this book is to provide you with a simple guide that will encourage you to make the right changes inside and out to achieve the health and wellbeing you deserve, to help you open your eyes to a different reality, or at least to create some curiosity about the benefits of a healthy body and mind.

Changing the way you eat doesn't have to be complicated, as you will see in this easy-to-follow guide. You will find a real food guide explaining how the quality of our food can affect our overall health and the impact poor quality food has on our systems. I also provide a list of pantry staples to keep on hand for healthy cooking. You will also find a healing foods section, which outlines the magical foods that acted as powerful medicine throughout my health journey. Then, the fun part: mouth-watering recipes that are simple and full of wholesome ingredients.

While my healing journey revolved heavily around changes in my diet, I learned that no matter how healthfully we eat, we cannot experience full healing unless we have a healthy mind, as mind and body are not separate entities. When my body suffered, my mind also suffered, so I had to learn how to protect my mental wellbeing in addition to my physical wellbeing. I will share a little more about my mental healing process in this book as well.

Looking back, I understand that everything happens for a reason. If I had never suffered from acne, depression, and other ailments for so many years, I would have never made these changes in my life. I would have never learned that food is our best medicine, and most importantly, I would not have had the chance to share my story with the purpose of helping you.

However, rather than simply trusting me, I hope you will trust yourself and listen to your body as you make decisions about your own wellbeing. No one knows your body like you do, so learn to tune into it. When you do, you will discover that it has the power to heal itself if you simply care for it and learn to love yourself.

Wishing you happiness and health all the way!

Introduction

Health: Your Most Valuable Asset

If I asked you what your most valuable asset is, what would you answer? Your car, your house, savings, family, friends or something else? What about your health? Did that answer even cross your mind?

Each person is unique; our ideas and values vary. We have different interests, responsibilities, and routines, but one thing that we all have in common, whether we realize it or not, is that none of us would be able to follow our passions if we didn't have our health. With a sick body, it becomes difficult to enjoy the best things in life. Health is priceless! Without health, we wouldn't be able to take care of our families, maintain a job, attend school or simply experience the blessing of being alive.

By being and feeling healthy, you can achieve anything, help others, and feel wonderful. Wouldn't it be nice to feel energetic and love your body every day? If you rolled your eyes at this last question, then let me tell you that it is possible. I can assure you from personal experience.

You Are What You Eat

It is inevitable that your body will start to react differently by changing what you consume. Your body only reacts to the treatment you give it. If you treat it well, it will thank you with good health, but if you don't take care of it, then it will start to deteriorate. Think of your body as being your pet. You have to feed it, allow it to sleep, relax, and exercise it in order for it to feel well.

The ailments we suffer, both big and small, are simply signals that our bodies use to tell us that something is wrong. Most people do not see acne or skin rashes as a sign that something is amiss inside their bodies. They also do not understand that depression is not simply caused by random chemical imbalances in our brains. All of the signs our bodies give us indicate that there is a problem with our system as a whole. Ailments are not isolated to the parts of our bodies that they affect, but are simply there to tell us to take a closer look at our overall health. Our bodies are meant to function like perfectly oiled machines and when they are properly taken care of, they will reward us with health and beauty.

So, how do we keep our system fueled and running at full speed? Can we use nutrition to achieve optimal health? According to my experience with chronic acne and several other ailments, the answer is yes! Our food is our fuel. We need the right fuel so our bodies can run efficiently. Imagine putting diesel in a gasoline vehicle— it simply won't run as well. The same is true for our bodies. If we eat low-quality food and don't take care of ourselves, then our health won't reach its full potential.

Why is it that we spend outrageous amounts of money on cars, clothes, and other luxuries, and often let our health fall to the wayside? Why do we spend more time watching TV or hooked on the Internet than using that time to cook our meals, exercise, or spend quality time with friends and family? After everything I went through, I learned that there is no better asset than my health and no better feeling than being healthy and energetic every day. I also learned that food is medicine and diet alone can optimize health.

This book will explain how food both heals and protects our bodies from disease. You will find simple and tasty recipes that don't require a chef's degree. The only requirement is your willingness to make some time for you.

Food Can Be Medicine

In our society, doctors are not trained to treat or prevent illness with nutrition; instead, they are trained to manage disease with drugs. In my opinion, this is one of the sole reasons why so many of us are sick—we don't know how to take care of ourselves. All we know how to do is mask our symptoms with pharmaceuticals, which interrupts our bodies' natural healing processes.

During my journey to get my health back, I had to learn that if I ever wanted to heal my condition permanently, I had to stop focusing on the symptoms and begin treating the root cause. As I have mentioned before, my main concern was acne, but I was also experiencing many other symptoms such as constipation, depression, insomnia, constant flues, and asthma, among other discomforts. I learned that I needed to focus mainly on healing my gut because the digestive system and the immune system are directly connected. Surprisingly, nearly 70% of our immune system is housed in the digestive tract. By eating right, we feed our bodies the nutrients, minerals and vitamins that are needed in order to maintain optimal digestive health, which in turn leads to a strong immune system. Our immune systems, when working properly, prevent us from getting sick and becoming hosts of viruses, bacteria and other pathogens that hurt our bodies.

Changing my diet was one of the greatest contributing factors to my body's ability to heal itself, but was also the greatest challenge. Yes, food can be amazing medicine, but we as humans are very emotionally attached to it and changing the way we eat can be extremely difficult, and dare I say it, life-altering.

However, these changes do not have to be made in one day; they can be made incrementally. The most important thing you can do is educate yourself about proper nutrition and how to source quality ingredients. Once you know how food can positively or negatively affect your health and you start to feel the difference between eating well and eating poorly, you will not want to turn back. Also, eating right does not have to be a torture on your taste buds! I embarked on my adventures in the kitchen hoping to discover just that and I did, which is why I am sharing my creations with you.

I hope that learning about the benefits of eating real quality food, learning more about how diet helped me heal, and checking out these delicious recipes will encourage you to make nutritional eating a priority.

Real Food Guide

A ll food is like a powerful weapon. It can either be a powerful healing weapon or a powerful weapon of destruction. Nourishing food energizes us, restores us, and makes us feel our best. Poor quality food or foods we are intolerant or allergic to makes us feel lethargic and can lead to an abundance of health issues. It is poison to our systems.

Unfortunately, many of the foods we consume today, such as processed foods, do more harm to our health than good. While convenient and often inexpensive, processed foods lose their nutrients in the refining process.

Another reason our food lacks nutrition is because the nutrients in our soil have been depleted through over-farming the land and using chemical fertilizers and pesticides. Industrial farms use chemicals when raising plants and animals in their farming practices, which greatly affects their nutritional value.

So why is consuming nutrient-dense food so important? Well, nutrients in our food tell our bodies how to function. They give our bodies instructions and without these instructions, our bodies' processes are compromised. This excerpt from a popular textbook, *Perspectives in Nutrition* by Wardlow and Insel, explains just how essential nutrients from food are to our health.

"Nutrients are the nourishing substances in food that are essential for the growth, development and maintenance of body functions. Essential meaning that if a nutrient is not present, aspects of function and therefore human health decline. When nutrient intake does not regularly meet the nutrient needs dictated by the cell activity, the metabolic processes slow down or even stop."

This perspective on nutrition demonstrates that the food we eat determines whether or not our bodies will function at their optimal levels. Therefore, the way we think about food needs to change. Instead of counting calories or grams of fat, we should be asking ourselves, "Is this food nourishing for my body and promoting wellness?" While food can act as our enemy, it can also be our greatest helper and healer; we just have to understand how to allow it to work for us, rather than against us.

Now that you have an understanding of the importance of consuming nutrient-dense food, you may be wondering where to begin. What exactly is real food? Where do you find it? How can you guarantee its quality? I have compiled this Real Food Guide to help you through this maze. I can guarantee you that you will still have questions (probably a lot of them) after reading this but I hope that this spurs you to do more research and continue your quest to find the most nourishing foods available to you and your family.

Organic vs. Non-organic foods

The question of whether to buy organic or conventional food is like opening up a giant can of worms. I will try to give you as much information in a small amount of space as I can, but in short, organic is usually better quality than conventional food, and if you can afford it, you should buy it. However, there are several pitfalls that consumers encounter when it comes to selecting the best organic food. Here are a few of them:

- Organic processed foods: All processed foods, even if they are labeled organic, are still processed. This means they most likely contain preservatives, sugars, and other chemical additives that keep them from rotting on grocery store shelves. The FDA's standards on what products can be considered organic are not the most stringent, so be sure to read labels and limit your intake of any processed food, even if it is given the organic seal.

- Organic produce: The Environmental Working Group (EWG), a nonprofit organization whose mission is to "use the power of public information to protect public health and the environment" produced a shopper's guide listing the 12 conventionally grown fruits and vegetables that contain the highest pesticide levels. They are as follows (in no particular order): apples, strawberries, grapes, celery, peaches, spinach, sweet bell peppers, nectarines, cucumbers, cherry tomatoes, snap peas, and potatoes. EWG also created a Clean 15 list, which contains the conventionally grown produce items that are least contaminated with pesticides. The following fruits and vegetables are the safest conventionally grown crops to consume: avocados, sweet corn, pineapples, cabbage, sweet peas (frozen), onions, asparagus, mangoes, papayas, kiwi, eggplant, grapefruit, cantaloupe (domestic), cauliflower, and sweet potatoes. If you cannot afford to buy all organic produce, you can use this list to help you prioritize. Also, try to buy locally grown produce whenever possible. Because it is expensive to obtain a certified organic seal, many small farmers' produce is not certified organic, but they still use sustainable and/ or organic farming practices. Be sure to ask the farmer about his or her growing practices. Furthermore, locally grown, seasonal food tends to be much more nutrient-dense than food purchased at the grocery store because it has not traveled long distances and sat on store shelves for long periods of time.

- Organic dairy: Cows are meant to eat grass, not corn, and grass-fed cows produce healthier dairy products than corn-fed cows. Most mass-produced "organic" milk comes from cows that have been fed organic corn products, but not grass. So while organic milk is certainly better than conventional milk (which comes from cows that have eaten genetically modified corn), it is still not the best. Conventional and organic milk is also usually heavily pasteurized, which kills its beneficial organisms. Therefore, both conventional and organic milk lacks many nutrients that are only present in raw milk (read more about this in the "The Raw Truth on Raw Dairy" section).

Eat Fat, Be Thin

Low-fat diets used to be all the rage and now you're suddenly hearing that not all fats are bad. Because you're always hearing a different story, you may not know what to think. Fats are categorized by length and degree of saturation. Keep in mind that naturally occurring fats and oils are a mixture of saturated and unsaturated fats. There is not such thing of all saturated or all unsaturated fatty acids. Let me explain briefly the different types of fat based on their saturation levels. This will hopefully clear things up a little bit and make you understand that not all fats are made equal.

Saturated fats - These are the most stable types of fats and can be exposed to high temperatures without going rancid. Usually they are solid or semi-solid at room temperature. Saturated fats are found in tropical oils, such as coconut and palm oil, and animal fats like butter, ghee, lard, tallow, and bacon drippings.

According to modern diet guidelines, saturated fats are to blame for heart disease, obesity, nervous disorders, and diabetes, among other ailments. However, science shows that the actual villains are partially hydrogenated oils (like canola, vegetable, corn oils and others), which contain trans fats. Trans fats are loaded with free radicals, which can cause damage and inflammation in different parts of the body. Therefore, it is crucial to avoid any hydrogenated oils. Also, keep in mind that excess of sugar, in particular fructose (not the one found in fruit, but the artificial form like high fructose corn syrup) can lead to the health problems just mentioned.

Humans need saturated fats in order to maintain optimal health. Saturated fats boost our immune system, act as anti-inflammatories, provide us with energy, and help our bodies metabolize food. They also play a major role in intercellular communication, which protects us against cancer. Saturated fats are also necessary for proper lung and kidney function and hormone production. More than half of the fat in our brains is saturated, and it is required for proper function of the nervous system. Saturated fats also contain essential vitamins A, D, E and K. This is just a brief list of benefits of consuming quality saturated fats.

Monounsaturated fats – These tend to be liquid at room temperature. Like saturated fats, they do not go rancid easily and tend to be relatively stable. Monounsaturated fats are acceptable for cooking at lower temperatures, but it is recommended to consume them in their natural state (unheated) to keep their health benefits intact. Examples are extra virgin olive oil, avocado oil, and flaxseed oil.

Polyunsaturated fats – They contain omega-3 and omega-6, which are essential fatty acids that must be obtained from the food we consume because our bodies don't produce them. The best sources are wild fish, fish oil and pasture eggs. It is very important to maintain a diet with balanced amounts of these fatty acids. Some studies point to a desirable ratio of at least twice the amount of omega-6s as omega-3s, but no more than 4 times as much.

Omega-6s can be found in most plant oils (canola, sunflower, safflower, sesame, soy, sunflower, and peanut), also in oat germ, wheat germ and rice bran. Rich sources of omega-3s are found in cold water fish (halibut, trout, salmon and cod), flaxseed and flax oil, chia seed and sea vegetables.

In the U.S. it is easy to consume more omega-6 than omega-3 because of the large consumption of the plant oils mentioned above. Too much omega-6 encourage our body to engage in inflammatory responses such as constriction of blood vessels, clumping of blood platelets and other unwanted chronic inflammatory reactions. A correct balance of these two essential fatty acids is extremely important because it determines the flexibility of the cell membranes, which are in charge of almost all chemical communication in the body.

Polyunsaturated fats go rancid easily when exposed to heat and oxygen, therefore they should never be used for cooking. Refined vegetable oils, such as soybean, canola, sunflower seed, corn, cottonseed oil and margarine (made with vegetable oil) are the ones to be wary of. These rancid, oxidized oils have a very high content of omega 6, which can cause inflammation. They are bleached and deodorized in order to be sold and during the refining process they are exposed to high temperatures and oxygen leading to the creation of free radicals. The free radicals in these fats attack cell membranes and red blood cells, which can also cause inflammation throughout your body.

Refined vegetable oils have been proven to contribute to increased cancer, heart disease and many other ailments, such as digestive disorders, systematic inflammation, weight gain, osteoporosis, damage to the liver, and more.

A word on Cholesterol:

There are many misconceptions about cholesterol and its effect on our health. Many people believe that a diet that is high in saturated fats causes high cholesterol, which can lead to heart disease. However, what we eat only partially affects our body's levels of cholesterol because our bodies themselves produce 75% of our total cholesterol—the last 25% comes from food. Also, cholesterol is not always our enemy; we need good cholesterol to help our bodies function properly.

Furthermore, while cholesterol is vilified, it actually plays several important roles in our bodies. One of these is hormone production. During times of stress, we need more cholesterol to help our body make more hormones. It protects the body from free radicals in the blood and is a repair substance to heal arterial damage. Acts as an antioxidant and is a prosecutor of vitamin D - essential for healthy bones and nervous system, proper growth, mineral metabolism, muscle tone, insulin production, reproduction and immune system function.

Cholesterol produces bile, which works as detergent to break down the grease and assists digestion. Lack of bile produces bloating and prevents the absorption of essential vitamins A, D, E and K. Mother's milk is especially rich in cholesterol, which is essential for infants during their growing years to ensure proper development of the brain and nervous system.

What you need to watch out for is bad cholesterol, which turns into triglycerides (blood fats). Bad cholesterol is produced when we consume excessive amounts of refined carbohydrates, sugars, and alcohol.

If you are interested in learning about the importance of saturated fats and cholesterol to maintain good health, I suggest you read Know your Fats by Dr. Mary Enid or *Eat Fats, Lose Fats* by Dr. Mary Enig and Sally Fallon.

Grass-fed beef

Red meats have been blamed for causing two major plagues: cancer and heart disease. Interestingly enough, consumption of red meat has dropped in the United States in recent years, but both cancer and heart disease continue to increase at accelerated rates.

The real problem lies not within red meat itself, but rather, in the way it is produced. You may be surprised to hear that approximately two-thirds of beef cattle produced in the United States are given growth hormones and many are also given antibiotics. This is because factory farms only care about the bottom line and treat their cattle accordingly—as a commodity, not a living animal. The use of antibiotics on cattle is particularly dangerous, as this causes the spread of antibiotic-resistant bacterial strains. This spreads not only to other animals on the farm, but also to people who consume the animal products. Antibiotic-resistant strains of salmonella have been detected in the food supply already, demonstrating just how serious of an issue this has become. The combination of the use of growth hormones, antibiotics, and a diet of genetically modified grains makes for one unhealthy steak. However, properly and humanely raised cattle produce beef that is chock-full of health benefits.

Cows are meant to roam pastures freely eating grass, not corn or soy. When they are raised in this way, their meat is rich with healthy fats (Omega 3 and CLA), as well as tons of vitamins, such as A, D, B12, and minerals such as zinc, iron, magnesium, and copper.

Most of the animals raised under conventional systems have diabetes, cancer, arthritis, and other infections. When buying meat, remember that it is not possible to achieve health by eating sick animals.

Fish should be wild not farmed!

Fish and all seafood are rich in minerals, omega 3 fatty acids, and vitamins A and D, which are essential for optimal health. Consumption of high-quality seafood promotes healthy bone structure and protects us from degenerative diseases.

All these benefits can be found in wild-caught seafood. It is important, however, to consider the health of the body of water your seafood comes from. Since the earthquake struck Japan in April of 2011, nuclear radiation has been leaking from Fukushima and polluting the Pacific Ocean. Many studies have confirmed that this radiation contaminated much of the ocean's wildlife, making seafood from the Pacific unsafe to consume at this point in time. I suggest you do your own research and keep abreast on this unfortunate disaster.

Even though wild-caught fish can pose risks, farm-raised fish is almost always an undesirable choice. These fish are raised in polluted, crowded waters and fed antibiotics, hormones, grains and soy. As long as you make wise, informed decisions about the wild fish that you consume, it is a healthier option and tastes much better.

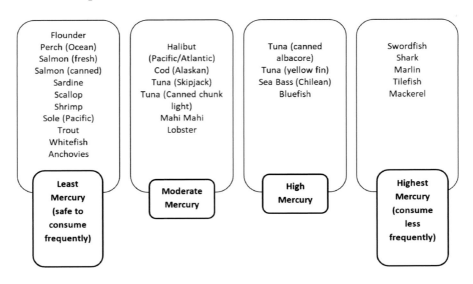

Flounder	Halibut	Tuna (canned	Swordfish
Perch (Ocean)	(Pacific/Atlantic)	albacore)	Shark
Salmon (fresh)	Cod (Alaskan)	Tuna (yellow fin)	Marlin
Salmon (canned)	Tuna (Skipjack)	Sea Bass (Chilean)	Tilefish
Sardine	Tuna (Canned chunk	Bluefish	Mackerel
Scallop	light)		
Shrimp	Mahi Mahi		
Sole (Pacific)	Lobster		
Trout			
Whitefish			
Anchovies			
Least Mercury (safe to consume frequently)	**Moderate Mercury**	**High Mercury**	**Highest Mercury (consume less frequently)**

The Breakdown on Sugar

In their natural state, sugars provide energy. Sugars and starches are supposed to be digested slowly and enter the bloodstream at a moderate rate over a period of several hours. This is not the case when refined sugars are ingested; to the contrary, they enter the bloodstream in a rush and cause sudden increase in blood sugar levels.

Do you ever feel tired or sleepy after a meal? The reason is probably because your body's regulation mechanism kicks in and releases large amounts of insulin and other hormones to help control its sugar levels. This happens if your meal is mostly composed of carbohydrates and starches (bread, whole wheat, rice, white flour, etc.). A few pages from here you will find a chart listing carbohydrates, fats, and proteins to help you decipher which foods fall into each category, which will help you balance your meals. If your sugar levels are constantly and drastically fluctuating, it can permanently damage your endocrine system and cause other problems such as diabetes and heart disease.

Refined sugars are found in almost every packaged food, sodas (regular and diet), commercial fruit juices, desserts, low-fat products, canned fruits, microwave foods, syrups, refined breads (including whole wheat), pastas, etc. This is why it is so important to make a habit of reading labels.

Artificial Sugar: Gravely Dangerous

In excess, refined sugar is certainly detrimental to our health. However, artificial sugars in *any* amount should be avoided at all costs. The most common artificial sweeteners you see in sugar-free and diet products are labeled as high fructose corn syrup, sucralose, aspartame, and acesulfame Potassium (commercial names include Equal, NutraSweet, and Splenda), which are worse than regular sugar. Keep in mind that anything that ends in –OSE is some sort of sugar.

Artificial and refined sugars have been linked to a broad range of diseases including diabetes, Candida overgrowth (a fungus in digestive tract that easily migrates to other organs), tissue and respiratory disorders, cancer, tooth decay, adrenal fatigue, blood acidity, and much more.

There are many more reasons why sugar should be consumed in limited quantities. It promotes the growth of tumors, damages and wrinkles the skin, and contributes to obesity and osteoporosis. When the body's blood sugar level drastically fluctuates on a consistent basis, the immune system is weakened, making us more susceptible to viruses, bacteria, and other pathogens. Excess sugar can also contribute to skin disorders, such as eczema and acne.

Sugar can be as addictive as any other type of drug. For me, limiting my sugar intake was one of the biggest challenges, but well worth it. If you find yourself always craving sweets, then I suggest that you start reducing the amount you consume each day and increase your consumption of healthy protein and fats. It will take your body some time to adjust, but you will soon find that you crave sugar less often and feel energized without it.

Nuts, legumes and grains

All grains, nuts, and legumes contain an organic acid found in the bran called phytic acid. Left untreated, this acid can block the absorption of essential minerals, such as calcium, magnesium, copper, iron, and zinc. However, when soaked or sprouted, these foods contain an abundance of health benefits.

Simply soaking grains, nuts, and legumes in clean, room temperature water reduces phytic acid so that the nutrients in the food are more easily absorbed. When grains, legumes and nuts are soaked, but mostly sprouted, this is what happens:

- Vitamin C production
- Vitamin B content is increased. Specially B5 and B6.
  - B5 – Pantothenic acid. Responsible for proper function of adrenal glands. Plays a vital role in cell metabolism and cholesterol production. Improves body's ability to deal with stress. Also found in organ meats and egg yolk.

- □ B6 – Pyridoxine. Helps proper function of over 100 enzymes. B6 deficiencies are common and are linked to diabetes, nervous disorders, and coronary heart disease.
- Breakdown of complex sugars, which can cause intestinal gas.
- Inactivation of a potent carcinogen called aflatoxins
- Production of enzymes that improve digestion

By simply soaking grains, nuts and legumes, you can minimize their nutritional inhibitors and maximize their health benefits. Soak overnight in filtered room temperature water with lemon juice, whey, sea salt, or other acidic medium. Discard water and cook.

For nuts, follow the same process then spread on a baking sheet. Dry at low temperature (less than 115 F) for 24-48 hours or use a dehydrator. Always be sure to dehydrate nuts at low temperatures, otherwise they will become rancid. Make sure to use raw nuts.

Eggs

Do not fear the egg! Eggs are rich in vitamins A and D, which are great for the skin and support the immune system. Eggs also offer high-quality protein that is filling and not stored in the body as fat. They are also loaded with lecithin, a substance that helps break down bad cholesterol and increases good cholesterol.

It pays to invest in high-quality pastured eggs, as conventional factory farmed chicken are fed genetically modified corn and soy and are often raised in inhumane, crowded conditions. The healthiest chickens should have space to roam and eat grass, bugs, worms, and non-GMO feed. Organic, pastured eggs are available at most health food stores. Their yolks are dark yellow or orange, indicating that they are much higher in nutrients than factory farmed eggs.

Pastured eggs are nutritionally superior to conventional eggs. Pastured eggs have more than three times the amount of Vitamin E and Omega-3s, more than double the amount of Vitamin A, and eight times the amount of beta carotene than conventional eggs.

Cooking destroys many of the nutrients contained in eggs, therefore, it is recommended to consume them raw when possible. Keep in mind that it is only safe to eat raw eggs if they are pastured, as they are much less likely to contain traces of salmonella. Poached eggs or soft-boiled are also good options if you choose not to eat raw eggs.

A note on egg allergies: Eggs are one of the most common allergens, however, most people are actually allergic to the white of the egg, not the yolk. If you do not have a serious egg allergy, try experimenting with egg yolks, which still contain an abundance of health benefits.

The Raw Truth on Raw Dairy

It took me by surprise when Shantih, my nutritionist, told me to add raw dairy to my diet. I was lactose intolerant for years and had to replace regular milk with soy milk, thinking it was healthier.... oh boy, was I wrong! Until then, I had only heard that raw dairy was dangerous and should be avoided at all costs.

After making changes to my diet and switching to raw dairy, I am no longer lactose intolerant. I have been consuming it for four years now and it has done wonders for my digestion, complexion, teeth, and immune system.

I understand that every person is unique and can also react differently to dairy. It is a matter of testing your body and seeing how you feel. When I started consuming raw dairy, I started with goat's milk, which is easier to digest; once I could tolerate it I tried cow's milk. It took my body a few days to adjust, but I soon noticed the wonderful health benefits of consuming raw dairy products. If you decide to give raw dairy a try, simply start with small quantities and monitor your body's reactions.

If someone does not tolerate raw milk it could be because of the lactose or casein content, but one thing to keep in mind is that in reality raw milk is not the problem, how well it is tolerated depends on the health of the digestive system. This concept applies to any foods, proper digestion and absorption depends on a gut functioning at optimum levels.

There are several factors that make commercially produced cow's milk dangerous and a highly allergenic food, which includes cows being fed an inappropriate grain-heavy diet, cows being treated with hormones and antibiotics, and pasteurization of milk. Cows are suppose to graze green pastures and eat hay in the winter months. Unfortunately, today's farming methods include feeding cows cheap, genetically modified soy and corn, which makes for unhealthy cattle and therefore unhealthy milk. Soy stimulates cows to produce larger amounts of milk leading to a high rate of mastitis. This type of feed also causes cows to suffer from liver problems, leads to sterility, and makes them prone to many diseases. In order to treat the diseases cattle are given antibiotics, which spread to the milk they produce. Hormones are also used to increase milk production in cows. These hormones not only negatively affect the health of the cow, but are passed down to the consumer through the milk.

Another factor that deteriorates the natural health benefits of milk is pasteurization. Raw milk is a living food full of beneficial bacteria, enzymes, and vitamins all of which are heat-sensitive. Pasteurization kills the beneficial bacteria in milk and decreases the bioavailability of the minerals making them harder for our bodies to absorb. This process is also what makes milk hard for people to digest. Enzymes present in raw milk including lipase, lactase, and amylase, are there to help our bodies digest it, but pasteurization kills these enzymes, rendering milk difficult for many to process. Many people who cannot tolerate pasteurized milk can tolerate and greatly benefit from the nutrients in raw milk, so it is worth exploring.

If you are highly lactose intolerant, it might be best to try fermented dairy, such as raw kefir or yogurt. Raw fermented dairy is virtually lactose-free because during the fermentation process the bacteria feeds from lactose. This is why raw kefir and other types of fermented dairy can be well tolerated by people who cannot digest fresh raw milk. These type products, particularly kefir, contain a lot of beneficial probiotics, which aid in digestive health. Even if you are able to tolerate raw milk, I recommend also consuming raw kefir and yogurt on a regular basis for added probiotic benefits.

Depending on the state you live in, you may be able to find raw milk and kefir at some health food stores. Regardless of where you live, you can always find certified farmers that produce raw milk and milk products in your area by visiting **www.realmilk.com**. If you are in California, I recommend you try Organic Pastures, they have a wide selection of high quality raw dairy.

Soy

There is controversy over the safety of soy. Soy contains phytic acid, which blocks the absorption of nutrients, including magnesium, zinc, copper, calcium and iron. While the phytic acid content in most grains and legumes can be greatly reduced by soaking or sprouting, this is not the case with soy. Instead, it has to go through a long process of fermentation in order to make it digestible. Therefore, it is only safe to eat in its fermented forms, such as tempeh, miso, soy sauce and natto.

Unfortunately, the majority of soy products on the market today are not fermented. Commercial soy like soy milk, tofu, soy protein powder, and soy baby formula are not only unfermented, but are likely to be derived from genetically modified soy. Between 90 and 95 percent of soy grown in the United States is genetically modified, so if you are consuming a nonorganic soy product, it is likely that it has been genetically modified.

There have been many studies showing that unfermented soy can be harmful to our health. Soy consumption has been linked to increased cases of breast cancer, cerebral damage, thyroid disorders, kidney stones, food allergies, infertility, debilitation of immune system, and more.

Always, make sure you read the labels of the products you buy because you will be surprised that soy sneaks its way into countless packaged foods in the form of soy lecithin, which is an additive. While I do not recommend consuming large amounts of soy lecithin, it does not pose the same health risks as soy and is relatively safe to eat in small quantities (ie: a piece of dark chocolate).

Life is better when you are healthy

When I first started changing my nutrition, I remember that I was spending lots of time at home submerged on the web, looking for recipes, beauty tips, and any testimonials that would lead me to believe I was headed in the right direction. I wouldn't eat anything outside of my house and restricted myself to an extreme level. I was very proud of myself for committing to changing my lifestyle, which was healing my body in ways that I never thought were possible, but it was also somewhat of a stressful experience because I couldn't really enjoy much of the outside world while being at home.

Balance is important; if you eat right 90% of time, then give yourself a break 10% of the time. By leading a healthy lifestyle, you are building a strong body that can handle something different once in a while. So don't be afraid to spend time with friends and family, travel, and do (or eat) what makes you happy. Enjoy your life—that's what health is for. Health allows you to see life from a different and better perspective. Trust that your body has its own intelligence and that by treating yourself right you are helping it perform its functions at optimal levels.

Proteins, Fats and Carbs Simplified

Below is a list of real foods broken down into categories. You may be pleasantly surprised to see that eating nutritious real food does not have to be bland or boring. Many of the foods you enjoy every day are probably on this list!

The daily amount of macronutrients recommended is 40% carbohydrates, 30 % protein and 30% fat. Everyone is uniquely made and therefore we have different nutritional needs, so monitor the way you feel and your energy levels after each meal, and adjust accordingly.

- **Protein**
- **Fats**
- **Carbohydrates**

MEATS

Meat is best if it is grass-fed, wild or pastured. Animals should eat what is closest to their natural diet in order to produce the healthiest meat.

Beef	Buffalo
Lamb	Elk
Pork	Venison
Chicken	Organ meats (liver, heart,
Turkey	kidneys, etc)
Ham	

SEAFOOD ●

Seafood is best if it is wild caught. Keep in mind that the list below does not include all seafoods available, so do not restrict yourself to this list. Please refer to the to "Fish Should be wild not farmed" section to see the chart that outlines the mercury content in various types of seafood.

Salmon	Mahi Mahi
Sardine	Shrimp
Tuna	Squid
Whitefish	Scallop
Bass	Lobster
Flounder	Oyster

DAIRY ● ●

Dairy is healthiest if it comes from pasture-raised animals and consumed raw or cultured. I also recommend choosing full-fat dairy products, as they are healthy fats. In the Healing Foods section, you will learn the importance of consuming raw and cultured dairy products.

Cheddar	Cottage cheese
Cream	Kefir
Cream cheese	Butter
Goat cheese	Ghee
Gouda	Yogurt
Milk (raw is better)	Whey
Parmesan	Mozzarella
Provolone	Sour cream
Swiss	Eggs (pastured are best)

NUTS AND SEEDS ●

Best if sprouted or soaked overnight and then dehydrated. Refer to the Real Food Guide section for instructions on how to soak grains, legumes, and nuts.

Almonds	Pumpkin seeds
Brazil nuts	Pistachios
Cashews	Chestnuts
Hazelnuts	Pine nuts
Flaxseed	Sunflower seeds
Macadamia nuts	Walnuts
Pecans	

OIL AND COOKING FATS ●

Keep in mind that these cooking fats have different smoke points, meaning that some are able to withstand higher temperatures than others without becoming rancid. Coconut oil, ghee, lard, and duck fat can withstand higher temperatures than olive oil and butter, so remember this when cooking.

Coconut Oil	Avocado oil
Coconut butter	Lard
Ghee (clarified butter)	Duck fat
Olive oil	Butter

GRAINS ●

Best if sprouted or soaked overnight. Refer to the "Real Food Guide" for instructions on how to soak grains, legumes, and nuts.

*High sugar (Eat in moderation)
** Very high sugar (Eat in moderation)

Basmati rice **	Barley *
Wheat products *	Buckwheat *
Brown rice **	Oats *
Wild rice	Quinoa
Cornmeal **	Rye *
Millet **	Spelt

LEGUMES ● ●

Best if sprouted or soaked overnight. Refer to the "Real Food Guide" section for instructions on how to soak grains, legumes, and nuts.

*High sugar (Eat in moderation)

Aduki bean
Black bean
Fava bean
Green pea
Lentil
Lima bean

Tempeh
Garbanzo
Navy bean
Pinto bean
Black-eyed pea*

FRUITS ●

*High sugar (Eat in moderation)
** Very high sugar (Eat in moderation)

Banana*
Cantaloupe*
Pineapple*
Watermelon*
Fig**
Date**
Raisin**
Prune**
Pomegranate*

Fruits with lowest sugar content:
Blackberry
Blueberry
Cranberry
Raspberry
and other types of berries

VEGETABLES ●

This list separates vegetables into *low, medium, and high* starch categories. Keep in mind that the body converts starches into sugars during digestion, so is best to consume vegetables that are lower in starch content. Generally speaking, high starch vegetables should be eaten in moderation; however, if you do intense physical exercise or are trying to gain weight, you can consume starchy vegetables more often if you do not have high blood sugar.

*High sugar (Eat in moderation)
** Very high sugar (Eat in moderation)

LOW STARCH	MEDIUM STARCH	HIGH STARCH
Broccoli	Eggplant *	Beet *
Brussels sprouts	Bell pepper	Corn *
Cabbage	Radish *	Potato **
Cucumber	Zucchini	Pumpkin **
Shallot	Avocado	Parsnip **
Tomato	Green bean	Yam **
Asparagus	Olive (all kinds)	Artichoke
Cauliflower		Carrot *
Celery		Summer squash *
Garlic		Sweet potato *
Ginger		
Mushroom		
Scallion		

Must haves in your kitchen

These are staples that I keep in my kitchen almost all of the time. Many of these ingredients make appearances in my real food recipes as well. Once you settle into your real food lifestyle, you will have a better idea of what you like to keep in your pantry on a regular basis and can keep it well-stocked.

Fats and Proteins

Organic coconut milk

I absolutely love coconut milk. It is so versatile, which allows me to use it in a variety of recipes. I can have it for breakfast, as a snack with fruits and nuts, and also use it in sauce recipes for dinner. It is a great replacement for milk and cream and makes a delicious base in hot chocolate and other creamy drinks for those who do not tolerate lactose. I prefer to use full-fat coconut milk because it is creamier and richer in flavor. Coconut milk has become increasingly popular and can be easily found at health food and regular grocery stores.

Virgin coconut oil

Coconut oil is one of the healthiest fats you can use for cooking. In the "Real Food Guide" section, you will learn about the benefits of consuming coconut oil, as well as other saturated fats. I like using unrefined coconut oil, which is the same as virgin coconut oil because it has anti-fungal and antimicrobial properties. It also is an excellent source of Lauric acid, which has great disease-fighting properties. Coconut oil has even more uses than coconut milk, as it can also be used for body care as massage oil, moisturizer, shaving cream, hair conditioner, and eye make-up remover.

Its uses are practically endless! You can find coconut oil at health food stores and grocery stores. This is a pantry staple that I definitely recommend keeping on hand all the time.

Eggs

Eggs from pastured chickens are the best option if they are available to you. However, they can be very expensive, so if they are not in your budget, organic eggs are also a good option and contain exponentially greater health benefits than eggs from conventionally raised chickens.

Kefir

I consider kefir a super food. It is most beneficial if made from raw milk from grass-fed cows. If you live in California, I recommend the brand Organic Pastures. You can also look for local farmers who may sell kefir at **www.realmilk.com**. This website provides a large list of certified farmers in your state. If you can locate kefir grains and raw milk, it is also easy to make kefir at home. Keep in mind that most store-bought kefir is made from heavily pasteurized milk and does not contain nearly as many beneficial strains of bacteria as homemade kefir. It also usually contains added sugars.

Grass-fed butter

Just thinking about butter makes me salivate! The best option is raw milk butter from grass-fed cows. If you live in California, I recommend Organic Pastures brand; otherwise, visit **www.realmilk.com** for certified farmers in your area. If you don't have access to raw butter, grass-fed butter is also a good option. I enjoy Kerrygold, which is available at health food stores and regular grocery stores.

Ghee

Ghee is a great alternative to butter for those who are lactose intolerant. Ghee is simply clarified butter, which is made by removing milk solids from butter. Therefore, it is lactose and casein free. Pure Indian Foods sells amazing ghee, which you can order online at **www.pureindianfoods.com**. **It is also easy to make your own.** Check out the recipe in the Healing Foods section below.

Cheese

I think I was a mouse in my past life — I am a fool for cheese! It can be enjoyed on its own, melted, or in countless recipes. It is preferable to buy cheese made from raw milk from pastured animals. If you cannot find raw milk cheese, aged cheese is also a good option. As cheeses age, their lactose content decreases, so you are less likely to experience ill effects that come from consuming pasteurized milk. Most health food stores offer a variety of raw milk and aged cheeses.

Bone stock

This is definitely a must-have in the kitchen. Using bone stock in your recipes will not only enhance the flavors of your dishes, but will give them an amazing health boost. You can learn to make your own (recipe in Healing Foods section) or there is always the option to buy pre-made bone stock at www.grasslandbeef.com or from a local store.

Grass-fed beef

Once you go grass-fed you never go back. The taste is unbeatable and the nutritional value is much higher than that of regular beef. Nowadays, grass-fed beef is becoming more popular and more easily accessible. The majority of health food stores carry grass-fed beef and even major grocery stores are starting to offer this healthier choice. There is also always the option to buy online or websites that help you find a local farmer who sells grass-fed beef. I find these websites reliable and trustworthy: **www.grasslandbeef.com** and **www.eatwild.com** If you can contact a local cattle owner, you may be able to buy a share of a cow, which is essentially buying beef in bulk, which ends up being much more affordable.

Organic chicken

I cannot emphasize enough the importance of the quality of the meat we consume. Organic, pastured chicken is tastier and more nutritional than conventional chicken. The best option is pasture raised chicken, although it can be expensive and trickier to find for some people. If pastured, organically fed chicken is in your budget, then that is the best option. Otherwise, organic chicken is a good choice as well. Pastured and organic chicken can be bought at most health food stores, major grocery stores, and online at **www.grasslandbeef.com** or **www.eatwild.com**. There are lots of online options, but these two are the ones that I had tried and feel comfortable recommending them to you. Again, if you can find someone who raises chickens and agrees to sell it to you, that is ideal.

Wild-caught fish

Not everyone is a fan of fish, but definitely make an effort to consume it once a week and make sure it is wild-caught to ensure that you are taking advantage of its nutritional value. Most health foods stores offer wild-caught fish and seafood.

Nuts

Make sure to buy raw nuts and soak or sprout them and dehydrate. They are perfect as snack, in yogurt or cereal for breakfast, and in desserts.

Carbohydrates - Fruits, vegetables and grains

Berries

Berries are a perfect addition to smoothies and parfaits, as snacks, desserts, or served with nuts or cheese. You can also buy frozen berries, as they tend to be a little cheaper than fresh berries, especially when fresh berries are not in season.

Unsweetened shredded coconut

Whenever possible buy organic, sulfate-free unsweetened shredded coconut. Shredded coconut can be used in smoothies, homemade snack bars, and in a variety of desserts. Most health food stores and major grocery stores sell it. I use it to enhance the consistency and flavor of my parfaits.

Avocados

These green beauties are extremely versatile. They are a great addition to salads, smoothies, and desserts. On top of their countless flavor pairings, they are a great source of healthy fat.

Most of the Naked Flavors recipes stick to the vegetables listed below. As many of you already know, organic is your best option if available:

- Tomatoes
- Onions
- Garlic cloves
- Cauliflower
- Bell peppers
- Mixed greens
- Mushrooms
- Lemons
- Cilantro
- Basil
- Zucchini
- Carrots
- Potatoes
- Sweet potatoes

Condiments

- Sea Salt (Himalayan or Celtic)
- Ground cumin
- Ground black pepper
- Powder garlic
- Crashed red chili peppers
- Dried basil
- Tomato paste (organic)
- Coconut Aminos (Tastes exactly like soy sauce, but contains no soy)

Alternative flours options

- Coconut flour
- Almond meal
- Cashew meal
- Arrowroot powder
- Tapioca flour

Healing Foods

I am a true believer that food is the most powerful medicine. How we feed our bodies can harm us, heal us, and even prevent us from getting sick. Regardless of how cleanly we eat, I learned that our bodies cannot fully heal without the boost that these healing foods provide.

When I first started to learn about the importance of eating real food, I consumed mostly organic produce, pastured and grass-fed meats, and clean water and noticed that I still was not seeing improvements in my skin, chronic fatigue, and other ailments. My functional specialist, Shantih, told me it was because my diet did not include healing foods, such as probiotic-rich fermented vegetables and beverages and gut-healing bone stocks.

You can eat the healthiest diet, but without these foods, your gut cannot heal. I had never even heard of some of these foods, and the tastes (ahem- sauerkraut) take a little getting used to, but I owe my success to these super foods. The probiotic content and gut-healing properties they contain do not compare to any supplement on the market. As these foods are not readily available in their most potent forms at the grocery store, you have to take the time to make them yourself and train your taste buds to tolerate them (well, not all of them— who doesn't love homemade chicken broth?!), but it is beyond worth it.

Surprisingly, after a while of consuming these healing foods, my skin began healing on its own and my digestion greatly improved. I actually began to enjoy these health tonics. After all, once you start noticing the effects these foods and drinks have on your body, it's hard not to enjoy them.

Kombucha

Kombucha is a probiotic drink full of live organisms that supports the health of your gut.

It helps boost your immune system, detoxifies your body, and gives you energy as it repopulates the good bacteria in your gut. The good and bad bacteria in our guts are constantly at war, and it is our job to make sure that the good bacteria always outweighs the bad in order to achieve optimal health.

There is plenty of information on the web about the importance of consuming probiotic foods on a daily basis. Kombucha is just one of a myriad of foods that is rich with beneficial microorganisms.

So what exactly is kombucha? It sounds strange, but it is actually just fermented tea. You have probably seen it on grocery store shelves, as it has recently become more popular and readily available. However, nothing beats the price and health benefits of the homemade version.

This ancient drink provides a large array of benefits. I have borrowed the following list from the handbook "How To Make Kombucha Tea" by Hanna Crum:

- Rich in probiotics – healthy bacteria
- Alkalizes the body – balances internal pH
- Weight loss – reduces sugar cravings
- Detoxifies the liver
- Increases metabolism
- Improves digestion
- Rebuilds connective tissue – soothes arthritis, gout, asthma
- Cancer prevention
- Alleviates constipation
- Boosts energy – helps with chronic fatigue

- Reduces blood pressure
- Relieves headaches and migraines
- Reduces kidney stones
- High in antioxidants – destroys free radicals that cause cancer
- High in polyphenols (plant chemicals that work as **antioxidants** to protect the cells in the body from free radical damage)
- Improve eyesight
- Heals eczema – can be applied topically to soften skin
- Prevents arteriosclerosis
- Speeds the healing of ulcers – kills h.pylori (type of bacteria that causes ulcers) on contact
- Helps clear up candida and yeast infections
- Aids healthy cell regeneration
- Reduces gray hair
- Lowers glucose level – prevents blood sugar spikes

When I started including kombucha in my daily routine, I noticed improvement of my bowel movements, a reduction in sugar cravings, (soda became a thing of the past), more regulated sleep, and my hair and nails began growing faster and thicker. Kombucha has become my morning drink, as it provides me with the energy I need to start the day.

After falling in love with this amazing drink, I began to pass on the word to my friends. Almost all of them admitted to seeing many of the same results I saw. However, one of the cases that truly surprised me was that of my friend Terry. She was addicted to soda (I am not exaggerating). She drank soda for breakfast, lunch, and dinner until one day the doctor told her she was likely to develop liver cancer and needed to reduce her soda intake. I suggested that she start drinking kombucha, and after a couple of weeks she had lost weight, felt more energetic, experienced better digestion, and most importantly, she was not craving soda anymore.

A few months later when Terry returned to the doctor for a follow-up appointment, he told her that her liver health had greatly improved.

I truly believe kombucha provides such an abundance of health benefits that it should be included in everyone's diet. If you have never had kombucha before, it is best to start with a small amount (4 -5 ounces a day for about three days). Listen to your gut—literally. If you feel good, then add another 5 ounces to your daily intake. I usually drink at least 16 ounces of kombucha every day.

Kombucha can be consumed any time throughout the day; if you drink it between meals, it will curb your appetite, and if you drink during or immediately following meals, it will assist with the digestion process.

If you are interested in learning more about kombucha, visit **www.Kombuchakamp.com**. This is one of the best online kombucha resources I have found that explains not only what it can do for your health, but also provides tons of tips on how to perfect the brewing process.

As I mentioned before, kombucha has become more popular and can be easily acquired at the majority of grocery stores. As your kombucha love grows stronger, you will notice that you are buying more and more bottles, which becomes expensive. Also, homemade kombucha is fresh, and therefore likely to contain more healthy strains of live organisms than the bottled versions that remain on the shelf for weeks. For these reasons, I make my own kombucha at home. It is very easy and you can make it in large quantities. See the recipe below.

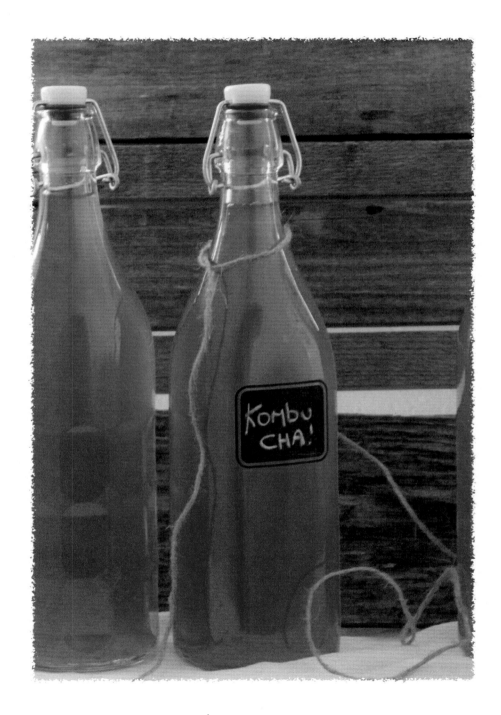

Kombucha recipe

Ingredients:

- 1 gallon glass container
- 3 quarts filtered room temperature water (make sure the water you use has no chlorine. It kills the live organisms that populate in the kombucha)
- 1 cup organic sugar
- 3 bags organic black tea
- 2 bags organic green tea
- 1 cup starter liquid (already made kombucha)
- 1 SCOOBY (You can find it online at **www.kombuchakamp. com**, Craigslist, or from your kombucha-obsessed neighbor)
- Kitchen towel
- Rubber band

How?

1. Bring one quart of water to a boil for a few minutes. Turn off heat and add tea bags. Let it sit for about 15 minutes.
2. Discard tea bags and add sugar. Mix until sugar has dissolved completely. Let it cool completely (this takes several hours). Note: Do NOT skimp on the sugar. The bacteria will not have enough sugar to feed on if you do not add the right amount of sugar, and therefore will not ferment correctly. By the time the kombucha is ready to drink there will be virtually no sugar left in it.
3. When the tea has cooled completely, add it to the glass container along with the remaining two quarts of water.
4. Add the starter liquid and gently place the SCOBY on top with clean, dry hands. Make sure the water is at room temperature; otherwise it will kill the SCOBY.
5. Cover with cloth and secure with rubber band.
6. Place the kombucha container in a dark, ventilated, warm place. The culture strives in warmth (your kitchen countertop should be fine).
7. Let it ferment for 7 to 10 days. Simply leave it alone for that period— do not disturb it.
8. After 5 days you can taste your kombucha by inserting a straw and taking a sip. It shouldn't be too sweet or too sour. You will notice a new film starts forming on top of the liquid, which are new organisms that are created during the fermentation process. This is normal, as it is a live drink. The extra SCOBYs that form can be used to make more kombucha, for beauty purposes, or can be donated to your soon-to-be-kombucha - obsessed neighbors.

Lacto-Fermented Foods

Fermenting foods has been a tradition in cultures all around the world for hundreds of years. During the process of lacto-fermentation, bacteria feed on starch and sugar in the food, which creates lactic acid. This acid protects the intestinal barrier from external pathogens that can compromise our health. Lactic acid is a natural preservative that allowed people to store foods for long periods of time before the invention of refrigeration. In addition to preserving food, lacto-fermentation creates beneficial enzymes and b vitamins, as well as various strains of probiotics.

One of the main probiotic strains in lacto-fermented foods is lactobacilli, which is a friendly bacteria that lives in our digestive, urinary, and genital systems. In her book *Nourishing Traditions,* Sally Fallon explains that the proliferation of the bacteria in fermented vegetables "enhances their digestibility and increases vitamin levels. These beneficial organisms produce numerous helpful enzymes as well as antibiotic and anticarcinogenic substances. Their main by-product, lactic acid, not only keeps vegetables and fruits in a state of perfect preservation, but also promotes the growth of healthy flora throughout the intestine."

When preparing lacto-fermented foods, is it essential to use quality ingredients (organic vegetables and fruits), filtered water, and sea salt. This will help the lactobacilli perform at their best. Keep in mind that lacto-fermented foods are not meant to be eaten in large quantities. I try to eat a spoonful of lacto-fermented veggies with every meal. Think of the phrase, "a little dab will do ya" when eating fermented vegetables, which is a blessing for many people, as sauerkraut does not exactly taste like chocolate cake.

Bellow you will find a couple of recipes that I follow from the book *Nourishing Traditions* by Sally Fallon. This is my cooking bible, as it not only has countless healthy recipes, but also contains a lot of valuable information about healing, nourishing foods.

Of all lacto-fermented foods, sauerkraut is the most well-known. It is easy to make, but pungent in taste if you are not used to it. So why do I eat it? Because it is full of enzymes, vitamins, minerals, and friendly bacteria that so many other foods cannot provide. I consider it more of a supplement than part of my meal since I only eat a spoonful at a time.

Sauerkraut recipe
(Makes 1 quart)

Ingredients:
- 1 medium cabbage, shredded
- 2 tbsp sea salt
- ⅓ tsp black pepper

How?

1. Mix all ingredients in a bowl. Press with your hands or with a wooden pounder for about 10 minutes to release juices.
2. Transfer to a quart-sized, wide mouth glass mason jar with an air-tight lid. The top of the cabbage should be at least one inch below the top of the jar.
3. Close jar very tightly and let sit at room temperature for about 3-4 days.
4. Transfer to refrigerator. It will keep for several months.

Tip: During warmer seasons, check on the sauerkraut after two days. The fermentation process is much faster in warmer conditions.

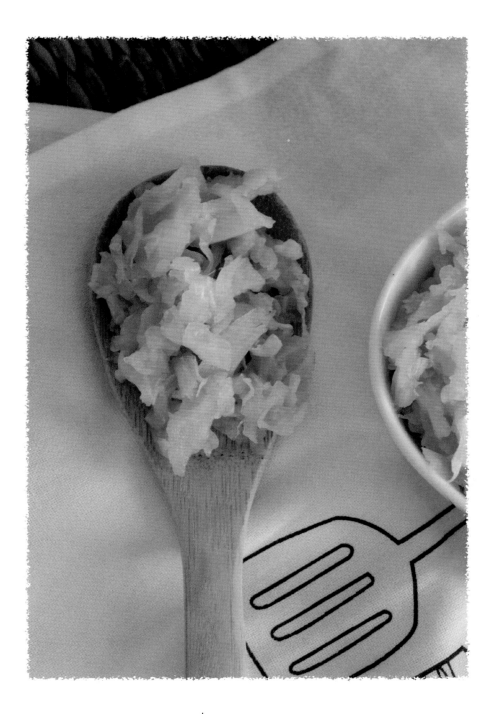

Bone Stock

Using bone stock for cooking not only adds flavor, but also a plethora of health benefits. Stocks are very nutritious when properly prepared and play a vital role in the gut healing process. Stock contains gelatin, which is rich with essential vitamins and minerals that boost the immune system, promotes healthy joints, ligaments, bones, and tendons, and protects hair and skin. Stock protects the digestive system from pathogens and has been used in the treatment of anemia, asthma, diabetes, and even cancer. Bone stock not only can improve health conditions, but also boosts the immune system when consumed on a regular basis to help protect the body from disease. I consume bone stock regularly to ward off even the sniffles, and it works like magic.

I learned about the miraculous health benefits of bone stock from some of the wisest experts in the field of natural health and medicine. In her book *Nourishing Traditions* (which I have now referenced several times), Sally Fallon writes, "Stock contains minerals in a form the body can absorb easily— not just calcium but also magnesium, phosphorus, silicon, sulfur and trace minerals. It contains the broken down material from cartilage and tendons— stuff like chondroitin sulphates and glucosamine, now sold as expensive supplements for arthritis and joint pain."

The list below comes from Dr. Mercola's website, which offers reliable and eye-opening health, nutrition, and lifestyle information. I highly recommend you visit his website.

Health Benefits of Consuming Bone Stock:

- **Helps heal and seal your gut** and promotes healthy digestion: The gelatin found in bone stocks is a hydrophilic colloid. It attracts and holds liquids, including digestive juices, thereby supporting proper digestion.
- **Inhibits infection** caused by cold and flu viruses, etc.

- **Reduces joint pain and inflammation**, courtesy of chondroitin sulphates, glucosamine, and other compounds extracted from the boiled down cartilage.

- **Fights inflammation**: Amino acids such as glycine, proline, and arginine all have anti-inflammatory effects. Arginine, for example, has been found to be particularly beneficial for the treatment of sepsis (whole-body inflammation). Glycine also has calming effects, which may help you sleep better.

- **Promotes strong, healthy bones**: bone stock contains high amounts of **calcium, magnesium**, and other nutrients that play an important role in healthy bone formation.

- **Promotes healthy hair and nail growth**, thanks to the gelatin in the stock.

(http://articles.mercola.com/sites/articles/archive/2013/12/16/ bone-broth-benefits.aspx)

In the five years that I have made bone stock a staple of my diet, I have only had the flu twice, and it was not severe. The consumption of bone stock has become more popular, especially for beauty purposes. People are realizing that it improves their complexions and beautifies hair and nails. I completely believe it because bone stock has done the same for me.

The way I include bone stock is by drinking a cup with every meal. I really don't mind drinking it plain, since it already is flavorful. I simply add a little bit of sea salt and squeeze some fresh lemon. When cooking grains and legumes I use bone stock instead of water.

You can sometimes find homemade bone stock at health food supermarkets, farmers markets, and online, but nothing beats the price of making bone stock at home. It is simple and requires little oversight. So here is the recipe if you are curious about this miraculous food.

Chicken bone stock recipe

Ingredients:

- 2-3 lb. organic bony chicken parts: necks, backs, wings, and feet if you can find them (the feet will increase the stock's gelatin content)
- 4 quarts cold filtered water
- Juice of 2 lemons
- 1 large onion, coarsely chopped
- 2 carrots, coarsely chopped
- 3 celery sticks, coarsely chopped
- 1 bunch parsley

How?

1. Fill a pot with filtered water.
2. Add chicken parts and vegetables.
3. Squeeze lemon juice and let it sit for 30 minutes to an hour.
4. Bring water to a rolling boil.
5. Cover and simmer for about 12 hours.
6. Once stock is done, turn off heat and let it cool completely.
7. Skim off the layer of fat. (This part is optional. I like leaving the fat in because it is flavorful and healthy for you.)
8. Transfer to containers and store in the refrigerator or freezer.

Tip: To make sure the stock has enough collagen, simply pour a little of stock in a cup and leave it in the refrigerator for a few minutes. If it acquires a gel-like consistency, then it is done.

For easy storage, pour two cups of stock in zipper storage bags or mason jars. Stocks will last for about a week in the refrigerator and several months in the freezer. If you decide to freeze make sure to use plastic containers or storage bags, glass will break. I learned this hard way!

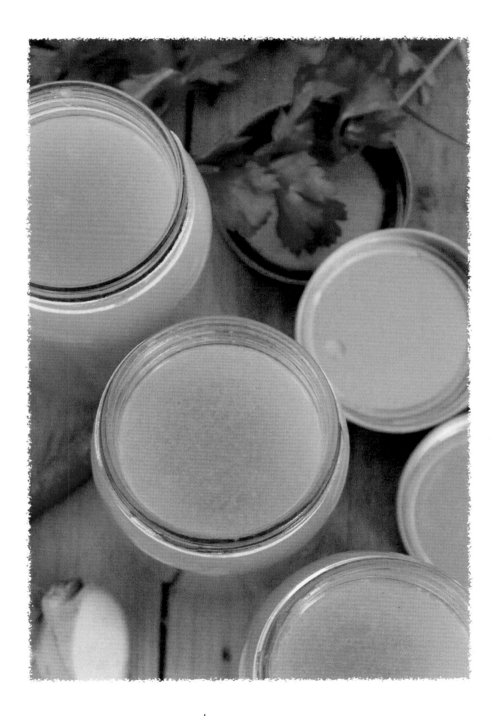

Organ Meats

When it comes to superfoods, organ meats are at the top of the list because of their incomparable content of vitamins and minerals that are often difficult to obtain in the diet. Organ meats boast a large amount of vitamin A, which is responsible for many functions in the body. In his website, www.mercola.com Doctor Mercola writes "Vitamin A is vital for prevention of birth defects, prevention of infection, hormone production, optimal thyroid function, good digestion, good vision, and healthy bones and blood. Without it, your body cannot utilize protein, minerals and water-soluble vitamins. Vitamin A is also an antioxidant that helps protect you from pollutants, free radicals, and cancer."

In addition to their high vitamin A content, organ meats contain iron, copper, zinc, choline (important for cell membranes, brain and nerve functions, heart health, and prevention of birth defects), vitamin E, CoQ10 (essential for energy production and cardiac function and also a potent antioxidant), and amino acids, just to name a few.

Even though there has been a lot of research done confirming the nutritional value of organ meats and that it is known that many organ meats are prized in traditional cultures as a crucial food to support vibrant health, our culture is not very familiar with these nutrient dense foods and we do not consume nearly enough of it. I could go on and on explaining the benefits of organ meats and how important it is to consume them at least once a week, but frankly it sometimes requires an open mind to give organ meats a try. Plus, it requires some preparation in advance to cook them.

If preparing organ meat is simply not an option for you (or you are working your way towards it), there is also a great supplement called Organ Delight by Dr. Ron's. These capsules are freeze-dried organs and glands that come from healthy, pastured animals. It is completely tasteless and uses only pure nutrients to achieve maximum absorption.

Homemade Ghee

Ghee is clarified butter that is both lactose and casein free. It can be used just like butter for sautéing, frying, as spread, in stews, or whatever you like! Like many healthy fats, ghee is resistant to high temperatures, meaning that it does not become rancid when heated and can safely be used for cooking.

When I first embarked on my healing journey, I was highly intolerant to lactose, so ghee was a great alternative to butter. As I mentioned previously, healthy fats are important for skin, joint, and overall health. You can find ghee at most health food stores or buy it online at **www.pureindianfoods.com**. It is also inexpensive and easy to make your own. You can use it to replace butter in any recipe.

Ghee Recipe

Ingredients:
- Cheesecloth
- Bar of grass-fed butter (Kerrygold is a great brand that you can usually find in the grocery store)

How?

1. Melt butter in a medium saucepan over low heat. Once the butter melts you will notice the clear fat will start to separate from the milk solids.
2. Continue simmering. Once it starts to bubble, you will know the water is cooking off. The bubbles will get smaller and will resemble foam. Milk solids will start to brown.
3. Keep a close eye on the pan. Once the milk solids turn a deep golden brown and start falling to the bottom (about 8 to 10 minutes after the melted butter starts bubbling), remove the pan from the heat.
4. Strain the hot ghee through a triple layer of cheesecloth into a heat-safe bowl, measuring cup, or directly into a glass container. Cool and store in refrigerator.

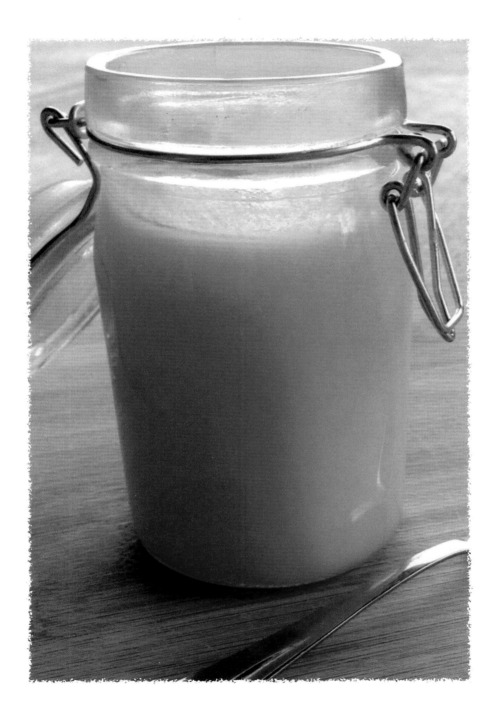

Recipes

Who said that eating healthy was boring? That's what I thought before I began changing my eating habits. I was under the impression that eating healthy meant eating tasteless, fat-free food, until I met Shantih, my functional nutritionist. He showed me a savory reality— real food has unmatched flavor, and even more importantly, real food heals our bodies and feeds our souls.

Nature is truly amazing; it provides us with all of the resources that we need to live a healthy life. Mother Nature ensures that every ingredient she provides has nutritional value and benefits our health. When you see food as your medicine, you not only enjoy it, but also come to realize that it is a blessing to be able to feed your body real food.

The process of changing my diet was a confusing and frustrating situation. I simply didn't know how to incorporate all of these seemingly obscure ingredients into my meals. First of all, I had to get in the kitchen and cook, which is something that I rarely used to do. Despite my lack of experience in the kitchen, I was determined to recover my health. I put my chef's hat on and pretended that I knew what I was doing. After burning food and some pots and almost setting the house on fire, I began to get the hang of it. With Shantih's recommendations and the help of several amazing blogs, I began to understand how to combine ingredients to thrill my taste buds and start to heal myself.

I now enjoy cooking, and my approach in the kitchen is to use real, simple ingredients that are easy to acquire. Most importantly, I am committed to incorporating ingredients into my recipes that are full of powerful nutrients, as this is how healing foods are created.

Always remember to cook with healthy fats at low temperatures, use quality ingredients, and take time to plan your meals so you can prepare them properly without becoming overwhelmed.

While eating, turn off the TV, leave your cell phone aside, and focus on savoring each bite. Never eat when you are under stress because your body secretes chemicals when you are anxious or stressed that can make food poisonous to your body. During my healing journey, I started to see mealtime as a sacred time. If I am alone, I meditate on my chewing, breathing, and the fact that I am grateful for the food I am fortunate enough to have. If I am dining with others, I use that time to engage in meaningful (but not stress-inducing) conversations. Mealtime is supposed to be a break in your day from whatever you are doing, so give yourself a break and savor every bite.

Allow yourself to be creative in the kitchen and don't feel confined to the ingredients in the recipes below— mix it up! If you feel there is something extra you can add or an ingredient that could be replaced, go for it! Experiment, play, and have fun in your kitchen!

Breakfast

Chia Pudding

Avocado Almond Bar

Egg Muffins

Flourless Bacon Pancake Dippers

Kefir Berry Smoothie

Avocado Smoothie

Choco-Banana Smoothie

Banana Pancakes

Apple Quinoa Breakfast Bowl

Mini Coconut Flat Bread

Tuna Omelette

Chia Pudding
(Makes 1 cup)

Ingredients:
- 2 tbsp chia seeds
- ¾ cup full-fat coconut milk
- ¼ cup kefir (preferably raw)
- 1 tsp maple syrup or raw honey
- ½ cup frozen or fresh berries
- 1 handful nuts

How?

1. Pour all ingredients into an 8 oz. mason jar.
2. Vigorously mix with a spoon.
3. Close lid tightly.
4. Let it sit for 10 minutes to allow chia seeds to gel.

Tip: This recipe is a great combination of fats, carbs and proteins (refer to Carbs, Fats and Proteins Simplified section to learn more). This is always a Favorite; family and friends love it because it feels so light in the stomach, but it's also filling. You can prepare several mason jars and place them in the refrigerator so you have breakfast or snack ready to go.

Many people use lack of time as an excuse for not eating healthy meals. An easy way to add healthy food to your daily routine is to prepare it in advance. In fact, you can prepare many recipes in this book in advance. Eating well is simply a matter of committing to it and organizing yourself to accomplish it.

Kefir can be replaced with yogurt (grass-fed would be ideal) or more coconut milk. If you're using only coconut milk for this recipe, make sure you add 1 more tablespoon of chia seeds to obtain the same thickness.

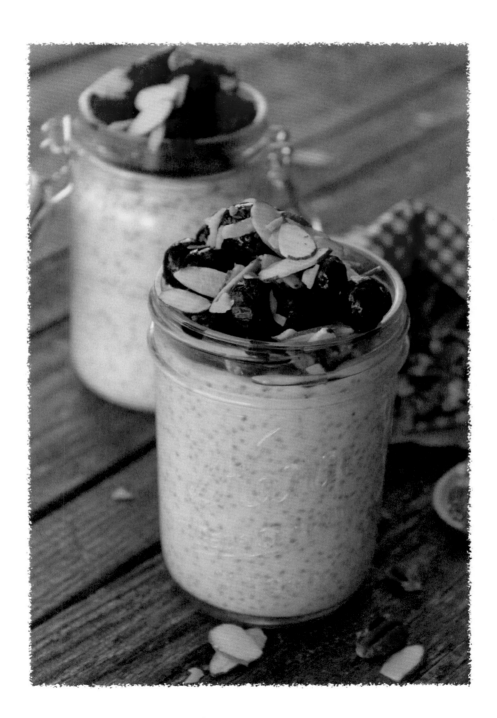

Avocado Almond Bar

Ingredients:

- 1 cup whole raw almonds
- 1 cup dried prunes
- ½ cup pumpkin seeds
- ¼ cup chia seeds
- ½ cup unsweetened shredded coconut
- 1 tbsp cacao powder
- 1 tbsp maple syrup or raw honey
- 1 medium avocado, mashed

How?

1. Place almonds and prunes in a food processor and pulse until a dough consistency has formed.
2. In a bowl mix pumpkin seeds, chia seeds, shredded coconut, cacao powder, and maple syrup.
3. Add this mixture to the food processor and continue pulsing for few more minutes until all the ingredients are blended.
4. Transfer "dough" to a bowl and mix with mashed avocado. You can use a spatula or your hands; I prefer using my hands.
5. Lay out a sheet of parchment paper, place dough on top, and cover with a second sheet.
6. Roll out to desired thickness with a rolling pin.
7. Freeze for 10-15 minutes.
8. Cut into bar size with a thin knife or pizza cutter.
9. Store in airtight containers or in a zipper storage bag and place back in the freezer.

Tip: These bars are delicious and really filling, which makes them great post-workout snacks. They usually last for about a week in an airtight container and longer if stored in the freezer, but I doubt they will last that long, at my house they disappear in a couple of days.

Feel free to replace whole almonds for sliced almonds, since they tend to be a little cheaper, and you can also substitute prunes for dates or figs.

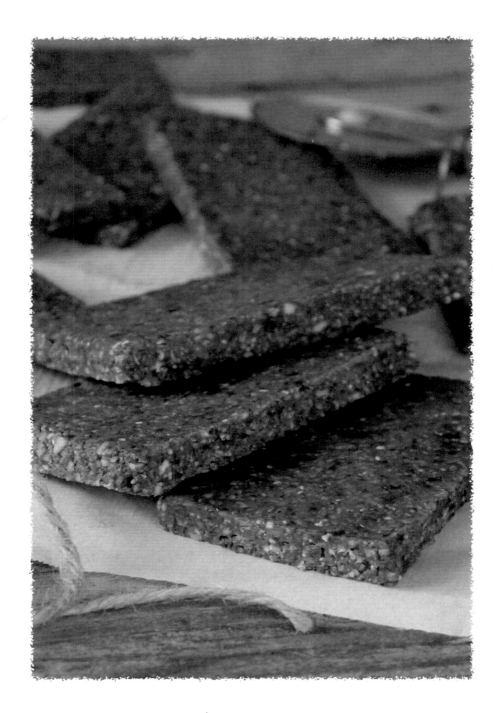

Egg Muffins
(Makes 4 muffins)

Ingredients:

- Coconut oil, butter or ghee for greasing
- 4 strips bacon
- 5 small mushrooms (crimini or white), quartered
- 3 eggs
- Sea salt and black pepper to taste
- ¼ tsp powdered garlic
- ½ tsp dried oregano
- 1 tbsp fresh basil leaves, finely chopped
- ½ tbsp grated parmesan cheese (or any other kind)

How?

1. Preheat oven to 350°F.
2. Grease a muffin pan.
3. Place each bacon strip around the inside of each muffin cup.
4. Fill each muffin cup with quartered mushrooms.
5. In a bowl, beat eggs.
6. Season with sea salt, black pepper, garlic and oregano.
7. Pour mixture evenly into each muffin cup.
8. Sprinkle with fresh basil
9. Bake for approximately 15 minutes or until eggs become firm.
10. Sprinkle with parmesan.

Tip: I like to take my time when I'm eating. I focus on chewing my food properly and enjoy every single bite, but I know that is not the case with everybody. So if you are always on the run these muffins are perfect to prepare in batches and store them in the fridge. That way you will have a nutritious breakfast waiting for you in the morning.

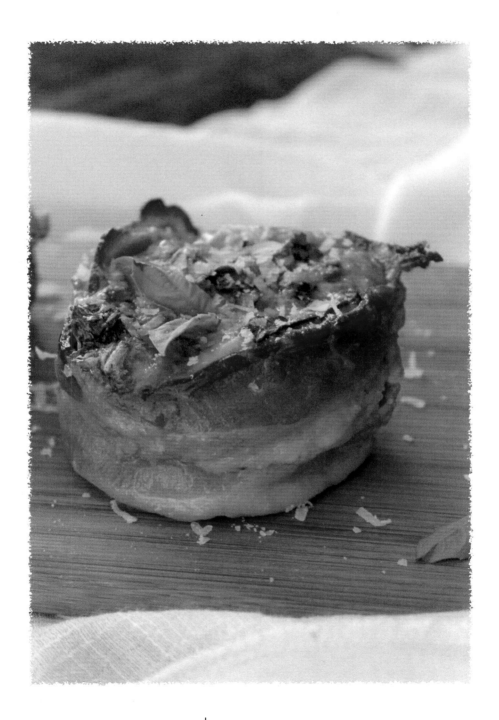

Flourless Bacon Pancake Dippers
(Makes 4 Dippers)

Ingredients:
- 4 bacon strips
- 2 tbsp coconut flour
- 2 tbsp coconut milk (full-fat)
- ⅛ tsp baking soda
- ⅛ tsp baking powder
- pinch of sea salt
- 2 eggs
- 2 tbsp maple syrup
- Extra coconut oil for cooking

How?

1. Cook bacon and set aside.
2. In a bowl whisk coconut flour, coconut milk, baking soda, baking powder, sea salt and eggs until there are no lumps.
3. In a pan melt coconut oil over low heat, add 1 tbsp of batter and lightly place a bacon strip on top. Cover bacon with a little more batter (less than ½ tbsp)
4. Cook for 1 to 2 minutes per side.
5. Repeat the process with the remaining pancakes.
6. Serve with maple syrup.

Tip: Wait! Don't flip the page yet! If you don't eat pork, you can still enjoy these pancakes. Just replace regular bacon for turkey bacon. I hope your tastebuds enjoy them as much as mine do!

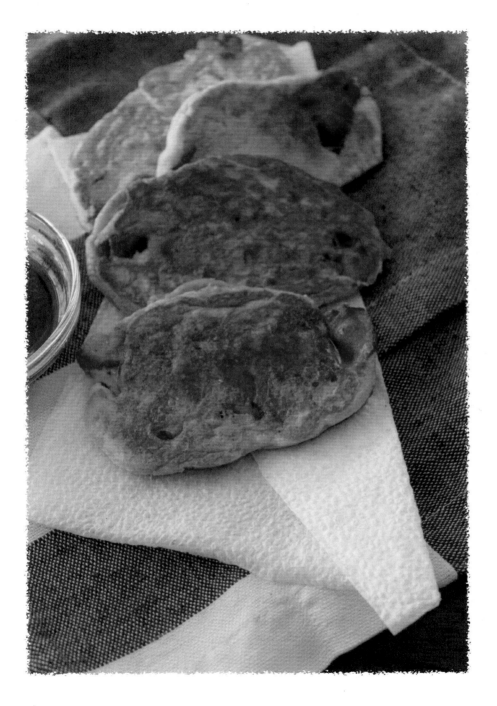

Kefir Berry Smoothie

(Makes 1 cup)

Ingredients:

- ½ cup full-fat coconut milk
- ¼ cup kefir (preferably raw)
- ½ cup berries, frozen or fresh
- 1 tbsp almond butter
- ½ tsp maple syrup or raw honey

How?

1. Blend all ingredients.
2. Enjoy!

Tip: Berries are your best choice of fruit because they are lower in sugar than other fruits. You can skip honey if you are using bananas or other fruits high in sugar. (Refer to the Protein, Fats and Carbs Simplified section to learn more about the sugar content in different fruits.)

The main reason I add raw kefir to my parfaits and smoothies is because of its rich probiotic content. Did you know that 1 tbsp of raw kefir has a least 60 strains and 150 billion bacteria? Amazing, right?

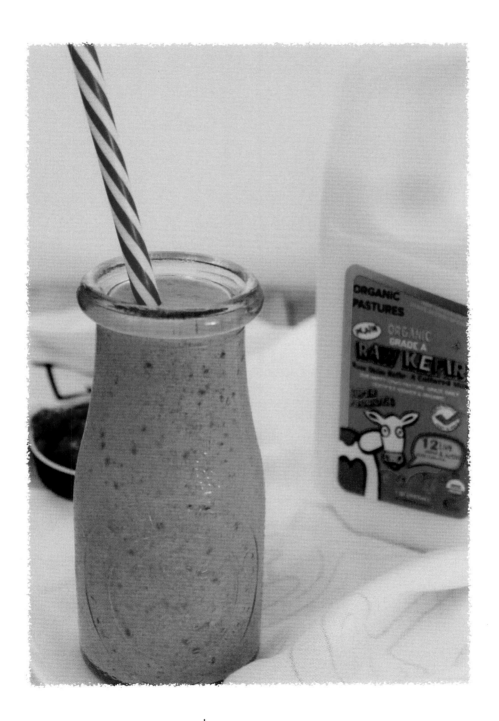

Avocado Smoothie

(Makes 1 cup)

Ingredients:
- ½ medium avocado
- ¾ cup full-fat coconut milk
- ½ cup crushed ice
- 2 tsp vanilla extract
- 2 tsp maple syrup or honey
- ½ tsp cacao powder

How?

1. Blend all ingredients.
2. Enjoy!

Tip: Feel free to adjust maple syrup and vanilla amounts according to your taste. This smoothie is really filling and keeps me satisfied throughout the morning.

I like to add raw cacao to my smoothies because I love chocolate, but also because of its magnesium content. Magnesium helps maintain healthy skin and a healthy nervous system, improves sleeping patterns, and much more.

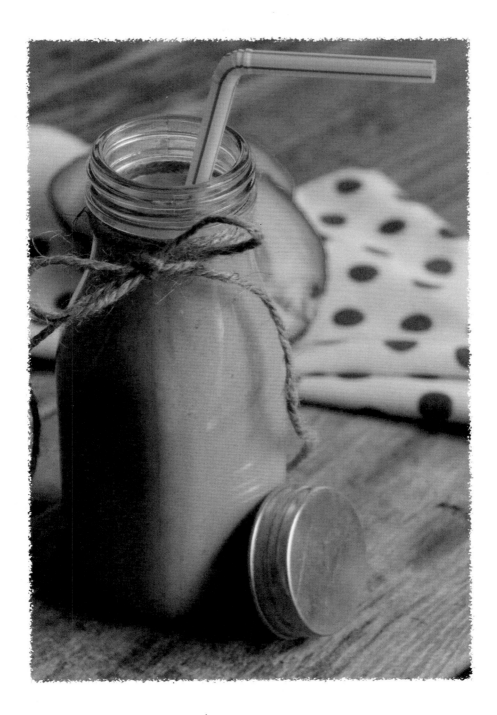

Choco-Banana Smoothie

(Makes 1 cup)

Ingredients:
- 1 frozen banana
- ¾ cup coconut milk (full-fat)
- ¼ cup ice
- 1 tsp maca powder
- 1 tsp raw cacao powder

How?

1. Blend all ingredients
2. Enjoy!

Tip: Maca is a Peruvian root that is mostly sold in powder form. Its distinct caramel taste is a great addition to smoothies or parfaits and it can be found at most health food markets as well as online retailers.

This superfood provides a wide range of health benefits: it is a hormone balancer, helps control the symptoms of menopause, and prevents mood swings. It is a great energy enhancer and a powerful aphrodisiac. It is definitely worth adding maca to your grocery list.

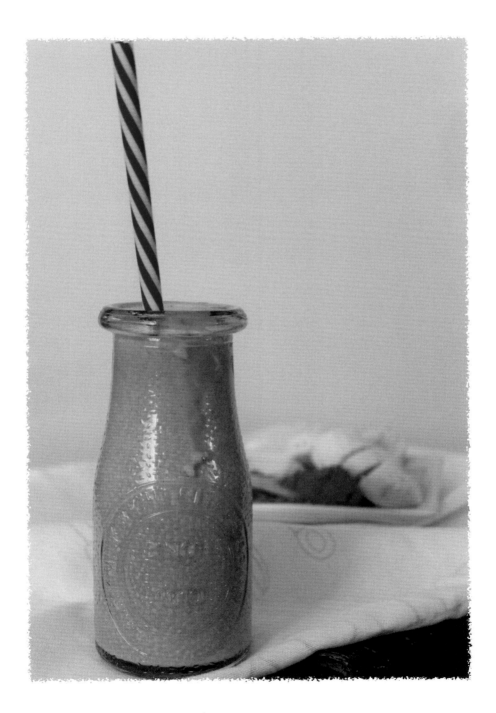

Banana Pancakes

(Makes 6 pancakes)

Ingredients:
- 2 bananas
- 2 eggs
- 2 tsp tapioca flour
- coconut oil for brushing skillet

How?

1. Mash bananas with a fork.
2. Mix mashed bananas with eggs and tapioca flour.
3. Melt coconut oil in skillet over low heat, spoon in batter, (approximately 3 tbsp of batter per pancake) cook for 1 to 1.5 minutes. Carefully flip pancakes and cook for another 30 seconds.

Tip: If you do your best not to waste food like me, then this is great recipe to use those overly ripe bananas that are about to have a sad ending in the trash can.

When I prepare these pancakes I like to top them with coconut whipped cream (recipe in Something Sweet section), yogurt (grass-fed would be ideal) or almond butter.

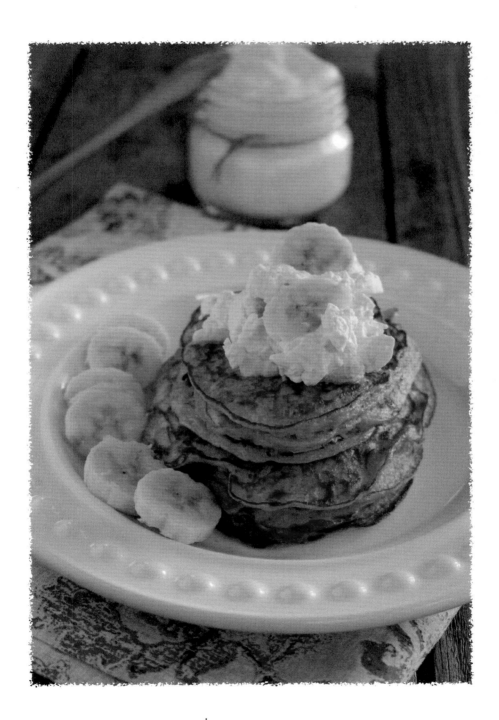

Apple Quinoa Breakfast Bowl
(Makes 2)

Ingredients:

- 1¼ cup full-fat coconut milk
- 1 small apple, chopped
- ½ tsp ground cinnamon
- 1 cup cooked quinoa (recipe in Sides section)

- 1 tbsp maple syrup or honey
- 1 handful of sliced almonds (or any other kind of nut)

How?

1. Heat coconut milk in a small pot over medium heat and add chopped apple. Cook for 5 minutes.
2. Add cinnamon and mix.
3. Add quinoa, stir and cook for 3 minutes.
4. Remove from heat. Add nuts and maple syrup. Mix and serve.

Tip: Make sure to soak quinoa overnight. This simple step will reduce the cooking time, but also it will prevent gas and bloating from happening. You can learn more about the benefits of soaking and sprouting grains, just look for the "Nuts, legumes and grains" heading under the "Real Food" Section.

Like the egg muffins recipe, you can also prepare this breakfast bowl in advance and store it in the refrigerator. It is to your benefit to have variety in your diet. One day you can have a breakfast with more protein and the following morning switch to a breakfast heavier in carbs, of course using grains properly prepared and if possible, fruits low in sugar content. This also applies to the other meals you consume during your day. (Go to Proteins, Fats and Carbs Simplified section to learn more about food categories). We are uniquely made and our bodies have different needs, but regardless, it is ideal to eat variety of foods to allow our systems to obtain all the nutrients it requires in order to work at optimum levels.

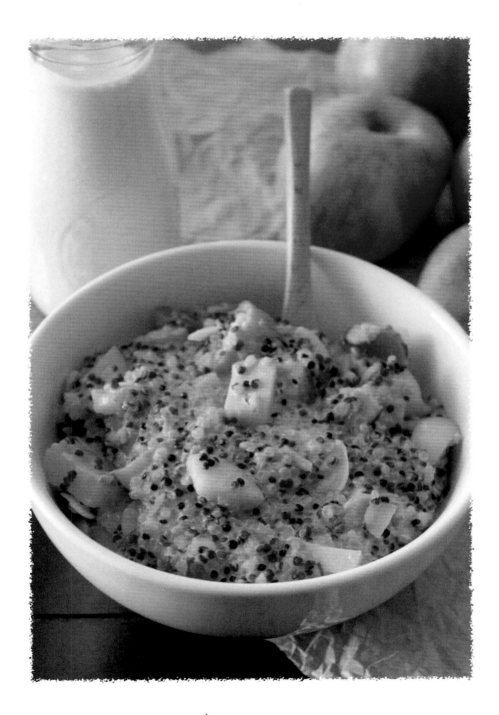

Mini Coconut Flat Bread

(Makes 10 small flat breads)

Ingredients:
- 3 tbsp coconut flour
- ½ cup full-fat coconut milk
- 3 eggs
- ¼ tsp baking soda
- ¼ tsp baking powder
- ½ tsp garlic powder
- ½ tsp sea salt
- ½ tsp dried herbs
- 3 tbsp coconut oil, melted
- Extra coconut oil for brushing

How?

1. In a bowl mix all ingredients and whisk vigorously until there are no more lumps.
2. Heat a skillet over low heat and brush with coconut oil.
3. Scoop 2 tbsp of batter for each flatbread. Let it cook until the edges start to brown and then flip (approximately 3 minutes per side).

Tip: Removing bread and sugars was one of the hardest things to do for me. These flats don't taste like a piece of toast, but are definitely a great option if you would like to have a sandwich. Here's an example of what I usually prepare: I place one piece of flatbread on a skillet over medium heat, top with cheese, slices of tomato, and basil. Cook for 2 minutes on each side or until cheese starts to melt. There are countless ways to spice up this bread, just let your creativity and taste buds guide you.

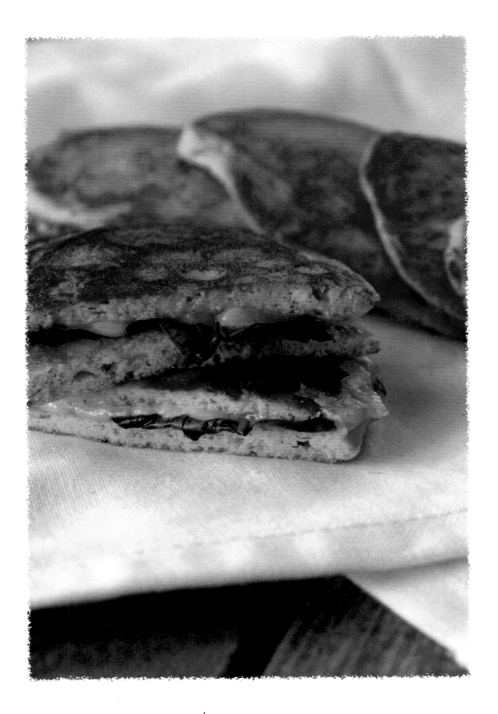

Tuna omelette
(Makes four omelettes)

Ingredients:
- 4 eggs
- 4 tsp full-fat coconut milk
- pinch of sea salt and ground black pepper
- 1 tuna can (wild caught)
- 1 tbsp fresh basil, finely chopped
- 1 tbsp homemade mayo (Recipe in Dressings section)
- 1 small tomato, sliced

How?

1. In a bowl beat 1 egg, 1 tbsp of coconut milk and season with sea salt and pepper.
2. Melt a little coconut oil, butter or ghee in a pan. Pour egg mix.
3. Cook for 2 minutes each side over medium heat.
4. Repeat the process with the remaining eggs.
5. In another bowl, mix tuna, mayonnaise and basil. Season with sea salt. Divide into four portions.
6. Spread tuna over half of the omelette, top with tomato and fold.
7. Repeat process for the other three omelettes.

Tip: When the body asks for protein early in the day, this a great way to satisfy that craving. Protein and fats provide us with lasting energy and makes us feel full for a longer period of time. Carbohydrates provide us with quick energy, but it lasts for shorter periods, which make our bodies crave food more frequently.

If you don't feel like using mayonnaise for this recipe, a delicious substitute is mashed avocados.

As you can see, all these breakfast ideas don't require too much time for preparation, even some of them can be prepared in advance to save you some time in the morning. I really hope these recipes show you that enjoying a healthy lifestyle is really not that hard.

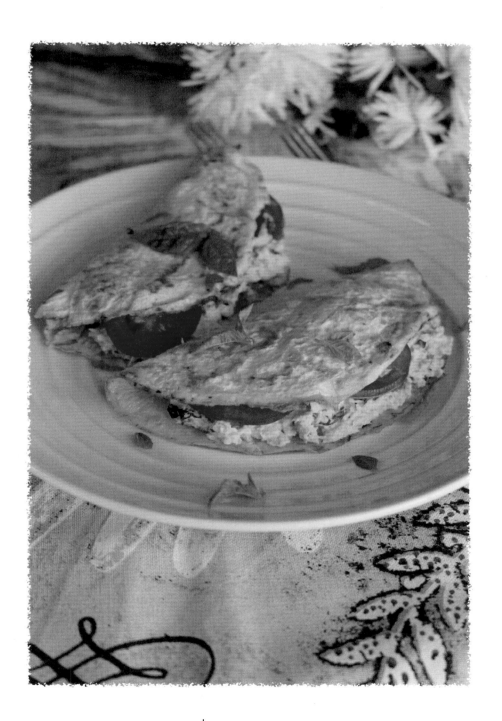

Beef

Korean Sirloin Steak

Lentil Chorizo Soup

Stuffed Bell Peppers

Zucchini Boats

Roasted Bone Marrow Spread

Cinnamon Beef Bowl

Korean Sirloin Steak

(Makes 3-4)

Ingredients:

- 1 lb. grass-fed beef sirloin steak
- ¼ cup coconut aminos
- 1 tbsp coconut sugar
- 1 tbsp toasted sesame oil
- 1 tbsp grated ginger
- 3 garlic clover, minced
- 3 tbsp butter
- 4 heads baby bok choy, halved lengthwise
- 2 tsp crushed red pepper
- 2 tbsp sliced green onions

How?

1. Score steak in a diamond pattern.
2. In a bowl mix coconut aminos, coconut sugar, sesame oil, ginger and garlic.
3. Place steak and bowl content in a seal bag and refrigerate for 6 hours or overnight.
4. In a pan, melt 2 tbsp butter over medium heat, add steak and cook each side for about 3 minutes for medium rare. I like to add a couple tablespoons of the liquid remaining in the seal bag. When flipping the steak try to place it on a different part of the pan.
5. Once steak has reached the desired doneness, place on a plate and let rest for 3 minutes so the juices get evenly distributed.
6. In the same pan where you cooked the steaks, melt 1 tbsp of butter over medium-low heat, add bok choy and cook for 2 minutes covered. Season with sea salt, pepper, crushed red pepper and green onions. Stir and cook for 2 more minutes.
7. Thinly sliced steak across the grain and season with sea salt. Serve with bok choy.

Tip: Why do I choose to eat beef medium rare? Amino acids remain almost intact when beef is not exposed to high temperatures for long periods of time.

Amino acids are the building blocks of proteins. We need constant supply of amino acids to be able to build proteins that provide structure to our bodies, such as muscles, nails, skin, eyes and organs. We are constantly rebuilding new tissue for example, red blood and skin cells last for about a month, cells of our intestinal lining last for two weeks. During times of healing we need more amino acids in the body to help regenerate of cells and tissues. Amino acids are also in charge to carry information from cell to cell and entire organ systems. In the Real Food section you will find more information about the benefits of consuming grass-fed beef.

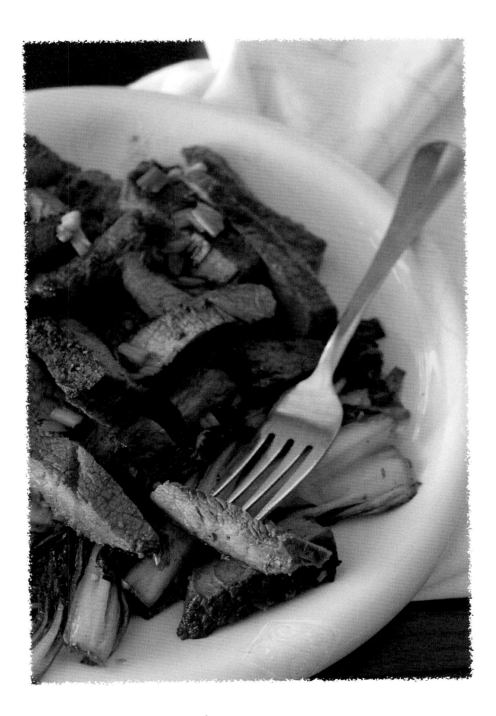

Lentil Chorizo Soup
(Makes 3-4)

Ingredients:

- 1 lb. hot pork Italian chorizo, sliced
- ½ tsp butter
- 1 onion, chopped
- 1 garlic clove, minced
- 3 scallions, chopped
- 2 tomatoes, chopped
- ½ tsp sea salt
- ¼ tsp black ground pepper
- ¼ tsp cumin
- 4 cups bone broth (chicken or beef)
- 2 medium sized carrots, peeled and sliced
- 2 medium sized russet potatoes, peeled and chopped into bite-sized pieces
- ½ dried cup lentils
- 2 tbsp fresh cilantro, finely chopped

How?

1. Soak dried lentils overnight in warm water with some lemon juice or sea salt.
2. In pot, melt butter and cook chorizo for 5 minutes, stirring occasionally. Once done, transfer chorizo to a plate.
3. To that same pot, add onion, garlic, scallions and tomatoes. Season with sea salt and pepper. Cook for about 10 minutes and stir constantly.
4. Add cumin and stir.
5. Add bone broth, chorizo, carrots and potatoes. Bring to boil for 5 minutes. Lower to medium heat and cook for 5 more minutes.
6. Add lentils and cook for 5 minutes or until lentils become soft.
7. Mix in cilantro and add sea salt and pepper according to taste.
8. Ladle into soup bowls and enjoy!

Tip: Every time you cook legumes and grains, make sure to soak just half of what the recipe calls for, otherwise you will end up with double the amount that you actually need. If you want to learn the benefits of soaking grains and legumes before cooking them go to the "Nuts, legumes and grains" category under the "Real Food Guide" section.

Not an oink oink eater? Feel free to replace pork chorizo with chicken or turkey sausage. If you'd like it to be a little spicy, simply add crashed red pepper to add a little kick.

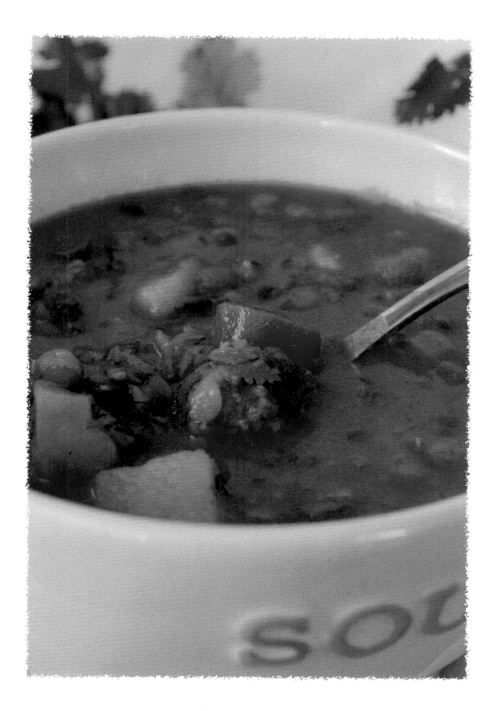

Stuffed Bell Peppers
(Makes 5)

Ingredients:
- ¼ cup raisins
- 5 medium bell peppers, any color
- Butter or ghee for greasing
- 1 tbsp butter or ghee
- 4 garlic cloves, minced
- ½ onion, diced
- 1 lb. grass-fed ground beef
- ½ tsp cumin
- ½ tsp ground cinnamon
- Sea salt and ground black pepper, to taste
- 1 tomato, diced
- 4 basil leaves, minced
- ½ cup shredded mozzarella or cheese of your preference

How?
1. Soak raisins in a bowl with hot water and set aside.
2. Preheat oven to 350°F.
3. Wash bell peppers, cut in half lengthwise, and remove veins and seeds.
4. Brush bell peppers inside and out with butter or ghee. Place them on an oven resistant plate and bake for 10 minutes.
5. Melt butter or ghee in a skillet over medium heat.
6. Cook garlic for a minute.
7. Add onions and cook until translucent (about 3-5 minutes).
8. Season ground beef with sea salt, pepper, cumin, and cinnamon.
9. Add seasoned beef to skillet.
10. Add tomatoes and basil.
11. Drain raisins and add to the skillet.
12. Cook on medium heat uncovered until beef is done, 5-7 minutes.
13. Once bell peppers are done, remove from oven and stuff them with the beef mixture.
14. Top each bell pepper with mozzarella or cheese of your preference and return to the oven for about 2 minutes.
15. Remove from oven and enjoy!

Tip: Oh boy! These stuffed peppers are so easy to make and are sure to be a crowd pleaser. I have made this recipe using dates instead of raisins and the results are still delicious.

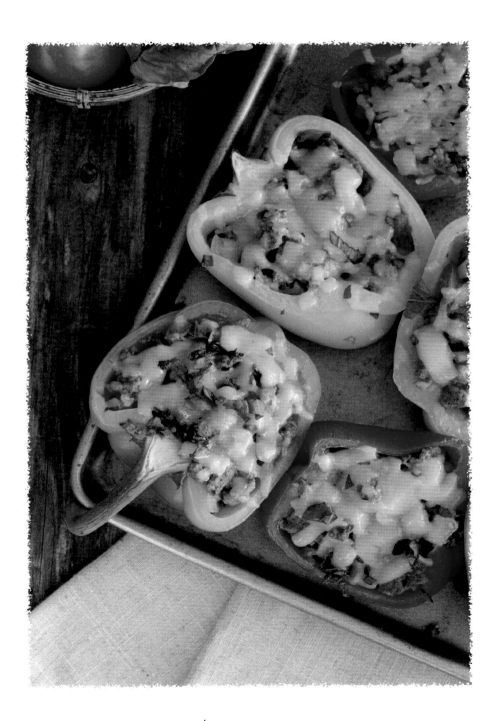

Zucchini Boats
(Makes 4-5)

Ingredients:

- 4 medium-sized zucchinis
- Butter, ghee or coconut oil for greasing
- 1 tbsp butter or ghee
- 2 garlic cloves, minced
- ½ onion, diced
- 1 lb. ground beef
- ½ tsp cumin
- 1 tbsp tomato paste
- 1 tomato, diced
- ⅓ bunch cilantro, minced
- Sea salt and black pepper, to taste
- 1 cup shredded mozzarella

How?

1. Preheat oven to 350°F.
2. Cut each zucchini in half lengthwise and scoop out the seeds using a soon.
3. Brush with butter, ghee or coconut oil.
4. Bake for about 15 minutes.
5. In a pan, melt butter or ghee over medium heat.
6. Add garlic and cook for a minute.
7. Sauté onions until translucent, about 3-5 minutes.
8. Add meat and season with cumin and tomato paste. Cook for about 5 minutes.
9. Add tomato and cook for 3 minutes. The point is not to overcook the tomatoes.
10. Toss in cilantro and mix.
11. Season with sea salt and pepper.
12. Stuff each zucchini half with beef mixture and cover with shredded mozzarella. Place back in the oven for a couple of minutes until mozzarella melts.

Tip: This is a simple recipe that is sure to satisfy most taste buds. If you prefer, you can replace ground beef for ground turkey.

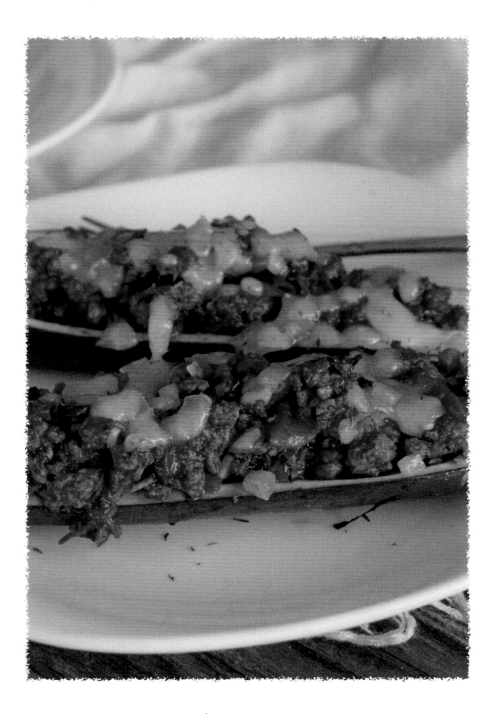

Roasted Bone Marrow
(Makes 2)

Ingredients:

- 2 lb. bone marrow (grass-fed), cut lengthwise
- ½ tsp butter or ghee
- 10 crimini mushrooms, coarsely sliced
- ½ tsp garlic powder
- Sea salt and ground black pepper to taste
- Dash of smoked paprika
- ⅓ cup shredded parmesan
- ¼ lemon juice

How?

1. Preheat oven to 350°F.
2. Roast bone marrow for 20 minutes.
3. In the meantime, melt butter in a skillet and sauté mushrooms for about 5-7 minutes.
4. Scoop out marrow with a spoon.
5. Place marrow, mushrooms, garlic powder, sea salt, pepper and paprika in food processor and blend.
6. Stuff bones with marrow mixture and cover with cheese.
7. Place back in the oven for two minutes.
8. Squeeze some lemon juice
9. Enjoy over quinoa patties (Recipe in Sides section) or sprouted toast.

Tip: Bone marrow is considered a superfood that not too many people talk about. It contains amino acids (building blocks of protein) that aid with digestion, assist in the healing of soft tissue and wounds, and helps maintain healthy skin and bones. Bone marrow also provides collagen, which has anti-inflammatory properties, protects the digestive tract from pathogens, facilitates digestion and assimilation of proteins. It is a great source of essential vitamin A, calcium, iron, phosphorus, zinc, selenium, magnesium and manganese.

Caution! Consuming bone marrow from chemical-laden cows will defeat the purpose because animals store toxins in their fat cells. So to obtain the miraculous benefits of this superfood it is important to choose bone marrow from grass-fed cows.

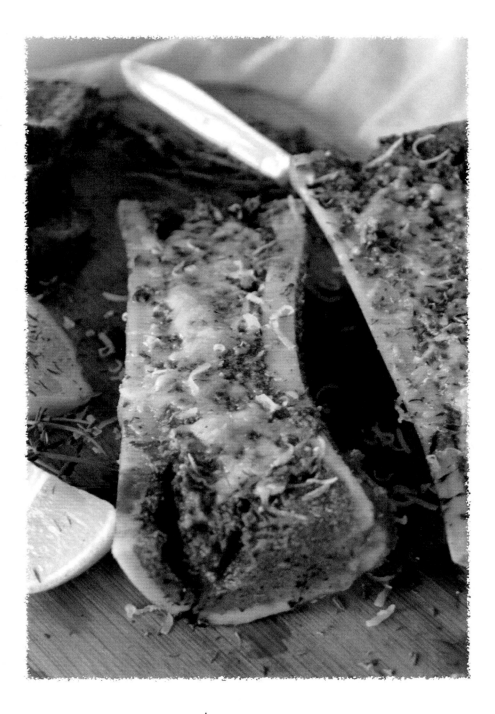

Cinnamon Beef Bowl

(Makes 3-4)

Ingredients:
- 2 tbsp butter
- 1 yellow onion, chopped
- 4 garlic cloves, minced
- 1 tomato, chopped
- 1 tbsp tomato paste
- 1 lb. ground beef
- 4 springs of thyme
- ½ tsp ground cinnamon
- 2 tbsp fresh cilantro
- 2 tbsp fresh basil
- Sea salt and ground black pepper, to taste

How?

1. Melt butter or ghee in pan over medium heat.
2. Add onions and sauté until translucent (about 3-5 minutes)
3. Add garlic and sauce for a minute. Then add tomato and tomato paste. Mix and cook for 3 minutes.
4. Add beef, thyme and cinnamon. Cook for 5-7 minutes.
5. Add cilantro and basil. Season with sea salt and pepper to taste and serve.

Tip: Cinnamon and beef? Weird, right? I thought the same too, until Clarissa, my sister from another mother, showed me how tasty it is to add just a bit of ground cinnamon to red meats. Give it a try and if you are not a fan you can always substitute with cumin.

A side of sprouted brown rice goes amazing with this meal. The butter and bone broth in the rice, brings this simple beef bowl to a whole new level. (Brown rice recipe in the Sides section)

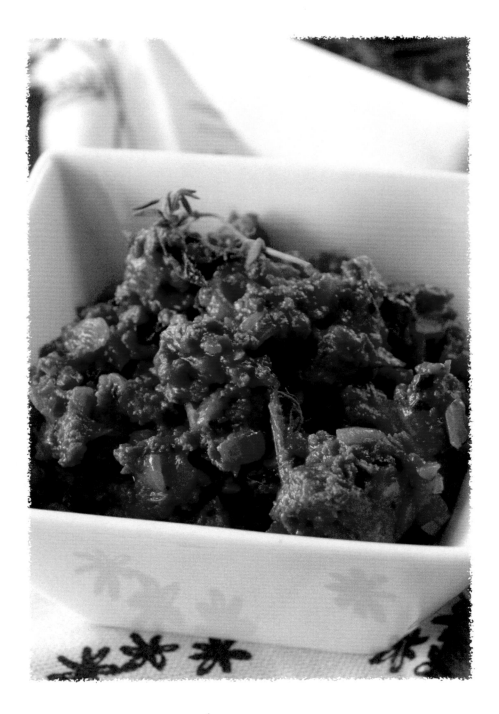

Chicken

Habanero Chicken

Chicken Estofado

Quinoa Chicken Bowl

Baked Chicken Drumsticks

Basilantro Chicken

Chicken Pot Pie Soup

You will notice that the recipes in this section call for chicken drumsticks and thighs. This is because organic, pastured boneless, skinless chicken breasts tend to be prohibitively expensive. Also, drumsticks and thighs are much juicier and more flavorful than chicken breasts. Feel free to use whatever chicken parts you prefer in the recipes below.

Habanero Chicken
(Makes 3-4)

Ingredients:

- 1 small habanero pepper
- 1 tbsp water
- 2 tbsp butter or ghee
- 1½ onion, chopped
- 3 garlic cloves, minced
- 1 tsp turmeric
- ½ tsp cumin
- 8 chicken drumsticks
- ½ tsp sea salt
- ½ tsp black pepper
- 3 cups chicken broth
- 2 cups of potatoes, diced
- 2 tbsp mint (chopped)
- ½ tbsp lemon juice

How?

1. Deseed habanero pepper and place in food processor together with water. Blend for a couple of minutes, until pepper gets liquified. Set aside.
2. Melt butter in a medium sized saucepan.
3. Add onions and sauté over medium heat until the onions are soft.
4. Add garlic and sauté for about 1 minute.
5. Add 2 tbsp of habanero pepper mix. Add more if you like spicy food.
6. Season with turmeric and continue to mix and cook for 1 minute.
7. Season all the ingredients in the pan with cumin.
8. Make small cuts on chicken drumsticks. Season with salt and pepper.
9. Add chicken and chicken broth. Cover and cook for 20 minutes.
10. Turn chicken and continue cooking for 10 more minutes.
11. Add diced potatoes and cook until potatoes are fork tender.
12. Add mint, lemon and adjust salt to taste.

Tip: These little habanero peppers and surprisingly spicy! This was my first time experimenting with them and because they are so tiny I thought they were mild—I was WRONG! When you are deseeding them make sure to wear plastic gloves or use a plastic bag otherwise your fingers are going to burn for couple of hours. No fun! I am not trying to discourage you from trying this recipe, it is just a word of caution.

This recipe was inspired by a traditional Peruvian casserole called Cau Cau. It is prepared with tripe, but I figured not everyone is a fan of eating intestines. So I used chicken instead and let me tell you, it is definitely worth a try.

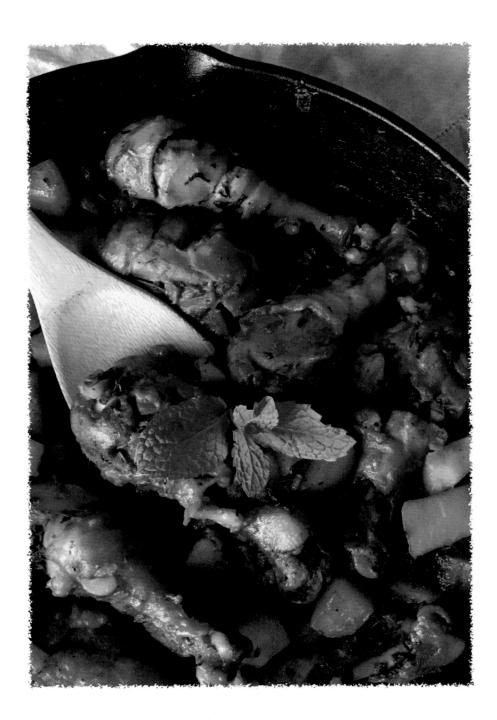

Chicken Estofado
(Makes 3-4)

Ingredients:
- 8 chicken drumsticks
- Sea salt and ground black pepper, to taste
- 1 tsp cumin
- 2 tbsp butter or ghee
- 4 garlic cloves, minced
- ½ onion, diced
- 2 tbsp tomato paste
- 1½ cup bone stock or water
- 4 medium Russet potatoes, peeled and diced
- 1 cup frozen peas and carrots mix
- 2 tbsp cilantro, finely chopped

How?

1. Season chicken pieces with salt, pepper and cumin. Cover and set aside.
2. Melt butter in a pot over medium heat.
3. Add garlic and cook for 1 minute.
4. Add onions and cook until translucent, about 5 minutes.
5. Add tomato paste and stir.
6. Add chicken and cook on medium for 5 minutes per side.
7. Pour in stock or water and cover. Cook on medium heat for 15 minutes.
8. Add potatoes and cook for 10 minutes.
9. Add carrots and peas and cook for about 5 minutes.
10. Add cilantro and mix.

Tip: I try to use bone broths or stocks (however you like to call it) for every recipe that calls for the use of water. Why? Well, bone broth supports the digestive tract, strengths the immune system by preventing external pathogens, such as viruses and bacteria, from entering the gut, helps seal leaky gut and also assist for better absorption of full proteins.

If you are in the market for beauty supplements, then bone broths are your best choice. Its high gelatin content gives the skin elasticity and prevents wrinkles, helps the growth of nails and hair. Since I started consuming bone broths on a daily basis, I have noticed that my nails growth faster and stronger and I don't mean to sound vain, but I love the way my hair feels and looks. If you want to learn how to make bone broths go to the Healing Foods section, they are super easy and cheap to make.

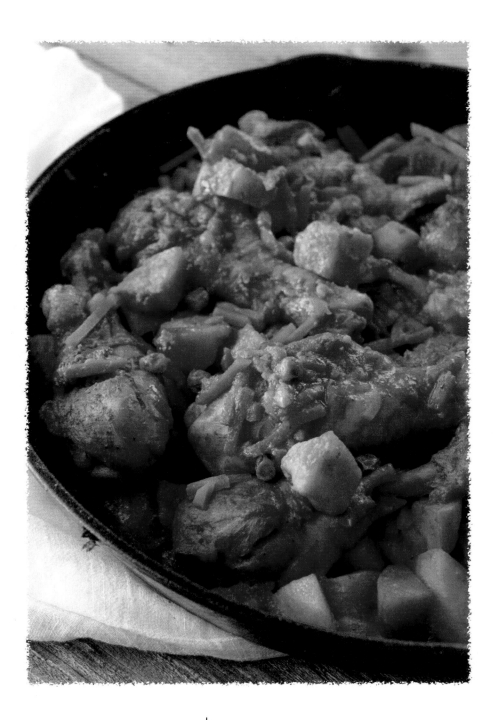

Chicken Quinoa Bowl
(Makes 4)

Ingredients:

- 5 bacon strips, chopped
- 1 garlic clove, minced
- ½ onion, diced
- 2 chicken breasts or 6 boneless thighs, diced
- Sea salt and ground black pepper, to taste
- ½ tsp cumin
- 1 tomato, diced

- 2 tbsp green onion, finely chopped
- 3 eggs
- 1 tbsp of butter, ghee or coconut oil
- 3 cups cooked quinoa (recipe in the Sides section)
- 1 tbsp coconut aminos

How?

1. In a pot over medium heat, cook bacon for about 2 minutes.
2. Add garlic and cook for 1 minute.
3. Add onions and cook until translucent (about 3 minutes)
4. Season chicken with sea salt, pepper, and cumin and add to pot. Let cook about 15 minutes, constantly stirring to prevent burning.
5. Add tomatoes and green onions and cook for 3 more minutes.
6. Beat eggs in a bowl and season with sea salt.
7. In a skillet, melt a little butter and cook eggs on each side for 3 minutes over medium-low heat.
8. Dice the omelet and add to chicken mixture.
9. Add quinoa to pot.
10. Season with coconut aminos and mix. Serve warm.

Tip: Remember to always soak grains before cooking. You can read more in the Real Food Guide, but to give you a summary. The main reason why it is important to soak grains and legumes is because all these foods contain phytic acid, which is an organic substance that plants use as a defense mechanism. This acid encapsulates all the minerals and vitamins found in grains and legumes. When this acid enters the body it makes it hard for the digestive system to absorb zinc, iron, phosphorus, magnesium, zinc and calcium. Eating grains without proper preparation can cause gas, bloating and inflammation and a frequent consumption of phytic can lead to vitamin and mineral deficiency, causing further disruption of our organs. Simply soaking raw grains and legumes overnight in room temperature filtered water with sea salt or lemon juice can reduce the amounts of this organic acid and make the nutrients found in these foods more readily available or absorption. This very simple step can make a positive change in your health.

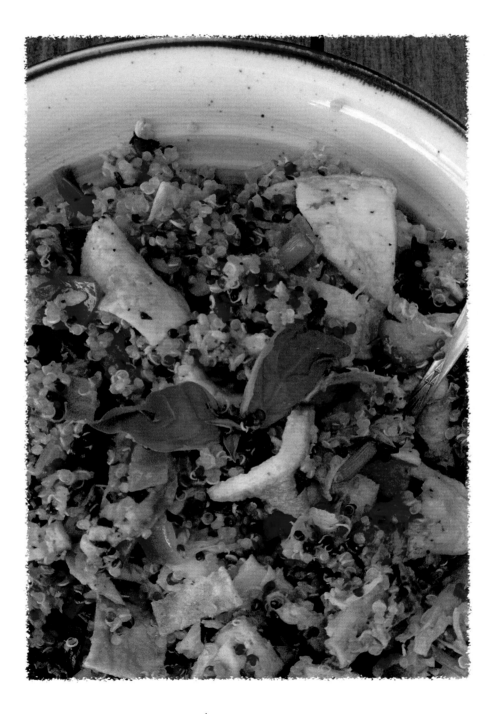

Baked Chicken Drumsticks

(Makes 4-5)

Ingredients:

- 8 chicken drumsticks
- 1 tbsp powdered garlic
- ½ tbsp cumin
- ½ tbsp sea salt
- 1 tsp ground black pepper
- 3 tbsp butter, melted
- 1 tbsp dried basil

How?

1. Preheat oven to 350°F.
2. Season chicken with garlic, sea salt, cumin and pepper.
3. In a bowl, mix melted butter with dried basil
4. Add chicken to bowl and rub butter all over chicken drumsticks.
5. Place chicken in a baking dish.
6. Bake for 45 minutes to 1 hour or until chicken is done.
7. Broil for 5 minutes.

Tip: If you decide to use chicken thighs the baking time will be less, approximately 25-30 minutes.

Do you ever have one of those days that you feel like doing…sh—er—nothing? If yes, then this is the perfect recipe for those days. I like to cook several drumsticks at once and keep them in the fridge, so I can have some protein ready to eat for whenever I don't want to make a big mess in the kitchen. I enjoy it in salads, sandwiches, soups of with any of the recipes in the Sides section.

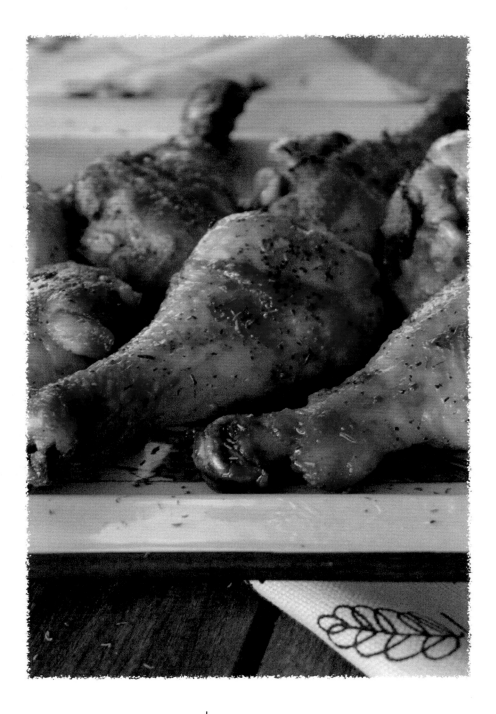

Basilantro Chicken
(Makes 4-5)

Ingredients:

- 8 chicken drumsticks
- 1 tsp cumin
- 1 tsp black ground pepper
- 1 tsp garlic powder
- Sea salt, to taste
- 2 tbsp butter or ghee
- 1 bunch cilantro
- 8 fresh basil leaves
- 1 onion
- 4 garlic cloves
- ¾ cup chicken broth or water

How?

1. Make small cuts on drumsticks and season with cumin, black pepper, garlic powder, and sea salt. Set aside.
2. Melt butter or ghee in a pot over medium heat.
3. Add seasoned chicken to pot and cook each side for 5-7 minutes.
4. In a food processor, blend cilantro, basil, onion, garlic and chicken stock or water. Season with a pinch of sea salt.
5. Pour content into pot and cover. Continue cooking on medium heat for 30 minutes and boil for 5 more minutes or until cilantro sauce has reduced.

Tip: The basil-cilantro sauce goes great with a simple side of sprouted rice or quinoa. I really recommend you to use chicken broth, as its flavor makes a big difference in the taste and consistency of this sauce.

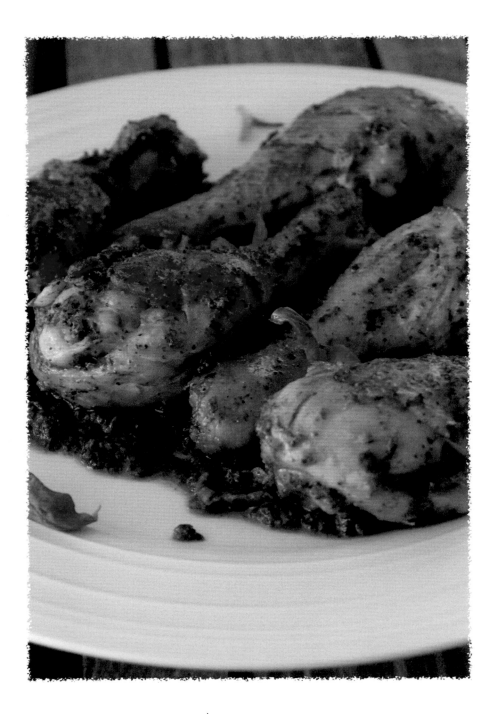

Chicken Pot Pie Soup

(Makes 4-5)

Ingredients:

- 5½ tbsp butter
- 1 yellow onion
- 2 chicken breast, diced
- Sea salt and pepper to taste
- 2 potatoes, cubed
- 2 cup chicken broth
- ¼ tsp dried basil
- ¼ tsp dried thyme
- 2 bay leaves
- 1 cup mixed veggies (green peas and carrots)
- 4 tbsp tapioca flour
- 1½ cup raw milk or any other milk you like
- ½ cup raw cream

How?

1. Melt butter 1½ tbsp in a pot over low heat.
2. Add onions and sauté over medium heat for 5 minutes.
3. Rub chicken with sea salt and pepper, and add to pot. Stir and cook for 12 minutes.
4. Add potatoes and chicken broth. Boil for 5 minutes and then simmer for 20 minutes or until potatoes are fork tender.
5. Press potatoes with a potato masher.
6. Add mixed veggies and cook for 5-7 minutes.
7. In a small pot melt the remaining butter over low heat and add tapioca flour, whisk and cook for about 2 minutes.
8. Add milk and whisk until there are no lumps. Add mixture to soup and season with sea salt and pepper to taste.
9. Add cream right before serving.

Tip: Raw milk can be replaced with coconut milk, just make sure it is full-fat. The taste will change, but if you like coconut you'll definitely love it. Also, tapioca flour can be replaced with arrowroot flour. And finally, if the soup is too thick or creamy for your taste, simply add more chicken broth.

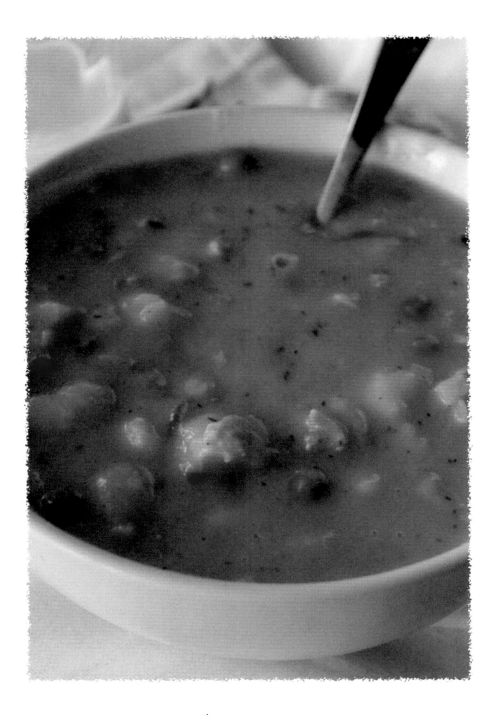

Fish

Sweet Lemon Salmon

Mushroom Salmon

Tuna Patties

Parmesan Lemon Cod

Lettuce Tuna Wrap

Sweet Lemon Salmon
(Makes 2)

Ingredients:

- 2 (6 oz) wild-caught salmon fillets
- Sea salt and black ground pepper, to taste
- 2 tbsp butter
- ½ tsp maple syrup or honey
- ¼ tsp dried thyme
- dash of garlic powder
- ½ tsp lemon juice
- Extra butter for brushing

How?

1. Preheat oven to 350 F
2. Season fillets with sea salt and pepper.
3. Squeeze just a little bit of lemon juice over fillets. Brush with a little bit of butter.
4. Transfer fillets to a cookie sheet covered with parchment paper and bake for 10 minutes.
5. In a small pan over low heat, melt butter.
6. Mix with maple syrup, thyme, garlic and lemon. Cook for 3 minutes.
7. Once salmon is done, place fillets in pan with butter mixture and rub on both sides.

Tip: If you are using frozen fish, make sure to thaw fillets before cooking and allow them to reach room temperature, otherwise they will have a rubbery consistency.

Another thing: when buying fish it is important to avoid farm-raised. Farmed fish is given inappropriate feed, such as soy pellets loaded with pesticides. Farmed raised salmon are dyed to make their flesh pink and its ratios of omega 3 and 6 are not as good as the ones found in wild-caught. Too much omega 6 in the body can lead to inflammation and consequently other health complications. If it is within your means, my sincere advice is to try to consume only wild-caught fish only. You can read more about the benefits of wild-caught seafood in the Real Food Guide section.

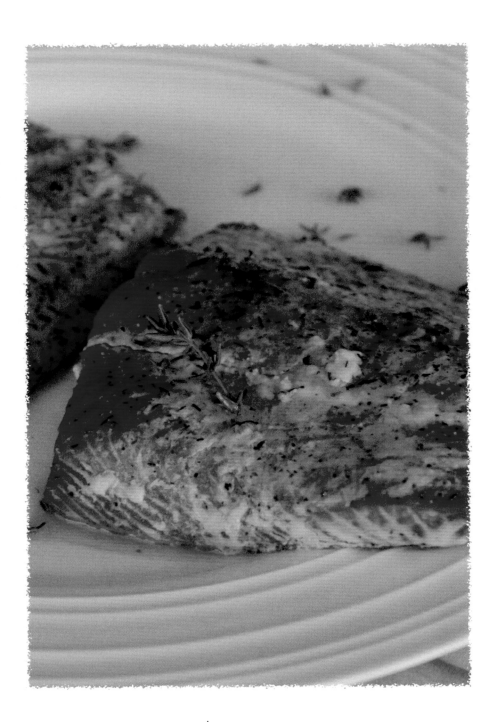

Mushroom Salmon

(Makes 4)

Ingredients:

*For fish:
- 4 (6 oz) wild-caught salmon fillets
- ½ tsp sea salt
- ½ tsp black ground pepper
- Butter or ghee for brushing

* For sauce:
- 3½ tbsp butter
- 4 tsp tapioca or arrowroot flour
- 1½ cup full-fat coconut milk
- 10 mushrooms (crimini or white), sliced (not too thin)
- 1 tbsp fresh basil, finely chopped

How?

Fish:
1. Season salmon fillets with sea salt and pepper.
2. Brush a skillet with butter and cook salmon over medium heat. Approximately 1½ minute per side.

Sauce:
1. In a pot, melt the 3 tbsp of butter over low heat. Add tapioca flour and whisk until there are no lumps (less than 30 seconds). Add 1 cup coconut milk and stir constantly.
2. Add mushrooms, ½ tbsp of butter and ½ cup of coconut milk. Cook for 3 minutes.
3. Add basil and stir.
4. Serve sauce over salmon fillets.

Tip: I like eating fish a little undercooked, but if you prefer to cook fish thoroughly, simply cook the fillets a little longer.

This is one of my favorite salmon recipes and it is always a winner when I cook it for family and friends. Give it a try. I am confident this salmon will thrill your tastebuds!

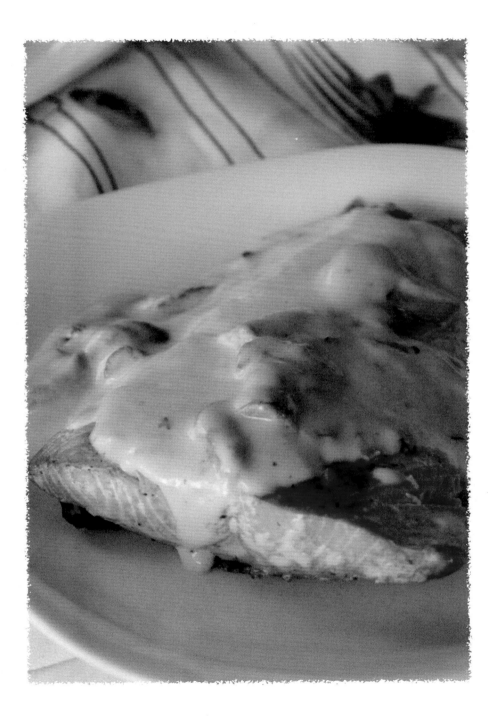

Tuna Cakes
(Makes 3-4)

Ingredients:

- 2 bacon strips
- 2 (5 oz) cans wild-caught tuna
- 2 eggs
- 3 tbsp cream cheese (preferably grass-fed)
- ¼ tsp black ground pepper
- ¼ garlic powder
- ¼ onion powder
- 4 tbsp fresh cilantro, finely chopped
- 2 tbsp fresh dill
- ½ small red apple, finely chopped
- 2 tbsp shredded parmesan cheese
- Sea salt, to taste
- Juice of half a lemon

How?

1. Heat a skillet over medium heat and cook bacon for 2 minutes each side. Once done chop into small pieces. Don't discard bacon fat.
2. Open tuna cans and drain out all the water.
3. In a bowl mix all ingredients listed, except lemon juice.
4. Form seven patties using your hands.
5. Cook patties in the same skillet you used to cook the bacon. Cook 3 minutes per side on medium-low heat.
6. Squeeze some lemon juice over patties and serve.

Tip: These tuna cakes go great with a side of sauerkraut or you can also have them in a sandwich. Simply spread some avocado or homemade mayo (recipe in Dressings section) on two slices of sprouted toast or quinoa patties (recipe in Sides section), add any desired greens and voila!

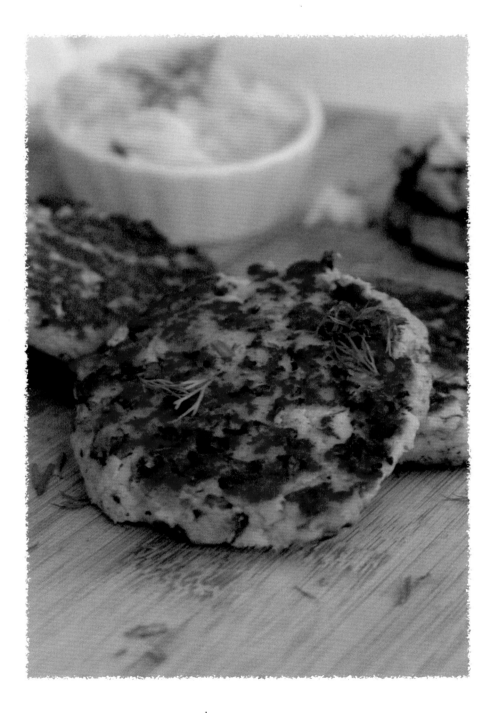

Parmesan Lemon Cod
(Makes 2)

Ingredients:
- 2 wild-caught cod fillets
- Sea salt and ground black pepper, to taste
- 5 tbsp grated parmesan (preferably raw)
- ¼ tsp garlic powder
- 1 tsp parsley, finely chopped
- Zest of ½ a lemon
- 2 tbsp butter, melted
- Juice of half a lemon

How?

1. Preheat over to 350 F.
2. Season cod fillets with sea salt and pepper.
3. On a plate, mix parmesan, garlic powder, parsley and lemon zest.
4. Set up an assembly line from left to right with fish, butter and cheese mixture.
5. Dip each fillet in butter and then in cheese mixture coating both sides.
6. Place fillets on a baking dish.
7. Bake for 10 minutes or until the fillets flake easily with a fork.
8. When done, squeeze lemon juice over fillets.

Tip: Honestly, I was never a fan of cod until I made this recipe. To me, cod tends to have a strong flavor, but when mixed with butter and parmesan cheese the taste is amazing! I hope you enjoy it as much as I do.

I always make an effort to consume fish once or twice a week because of all the exceptional benefits that it offers. Consuming fish promotes excellent growth and bone structure, it's a great source of macro and trace minerals, particularly iodine and zinc. Fish also is a rich source of vitamin A and D, which are essential for a healthy and strong immune system. In the Real Food Guide section you will find more information about wild caught fish and its health properties.

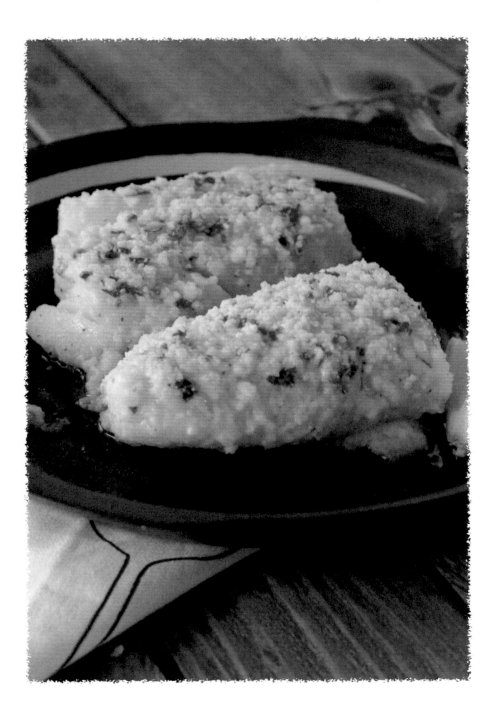

Lettuce Tuna Wraps

(Makes 4)

Ingredients:

- 2 (5 oz) cans wild-caught tuna
- 4 tbsp homemade mayo (recipe in Dressings section)
- 2 tbsp fresh basil, finely chopped
- 3 tbsp red apple, chopped
- 1 tbsp lemon juice
- Sea salt and ground black pepper, to taste
- 4 Romaine lettuce leaves
- 1 avocado, chopped
- 2 tbsp shredded parmesan cheese

How?

1. Drain out excess liquid from tuna cans and place in a bowl.
2. Mix tuna with mayonnaise, basil, apple and lemon juice.
3. Season with salt and pepper.
4. Spread tuna mixture on lettuce leaves.
5. Top with avocado and parmesan.

Tip: Life happens and sometimes we are stuck with work, school, and other activities that prevent us from cooking. However, there are countless options for real fast food. These wraps are super simple to make and are very filling, but it is better to eat them right away to prevent the avocado from turning brown.

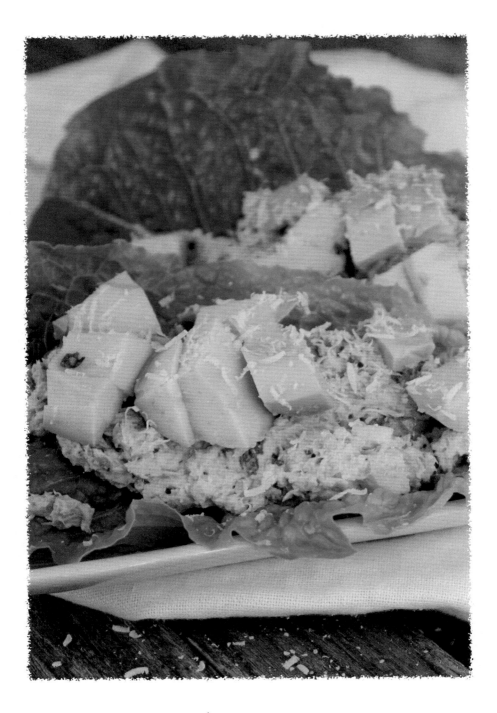

Sides

Quinoa

Brown Rice

Stuffed Potatoes

Bacon Brussel Sprouts

Quinoa Patties

Quinoa Pilaf

Sauté Green Beans

Cauliflower Tortillas

Sweet Potato Wedges

Tomato Avocado Salad

Quinoa
(Makes 2 cups)

Ingredients:
- 1 cup quinoa
- 1 lemon or ½ lime
- 1 cup chicken stock or water

How?

1. Rinse quinoa and soak overnight in filtered warm water with juice of one lemon or juice of ½ lime.
2. Discard water.
3. Add quinoa and chicken stock or water to pot.
4. Bring to boil for 5 minutes
5. Skim off foam and reduce heat to medium.
6. Simmer uncovered for about 15 minutes or until liquid has been absorbed.
7. Turn off heat, transfer to glass bowl and let cool for 5 to 10 minutes before serving.

Tip: The reason I like to transfer quinoa to a glass bowl right after it is done is to prevent quinoa from over cooking.

Simply soaking grains and legumes overnight makes a big difference in the body during the digestion process. Properly preparing grains and legumes helps the body breakdown the sugars found in theses foods, which can cause intestinal gas and bloating. By soaking or sprouting, the levels of vitamin C and B are increased. Why is this important? Because these vitamins strengthen the immune system, vitamin B helps our adrenals function at optimum levels and improves our ability to deal with any type of stress. So, do your gut a favor and soak grains before cooking. Plus, you'll also be helping your wallet because after soaking, the grains puff up and and give you more bang for your buck!

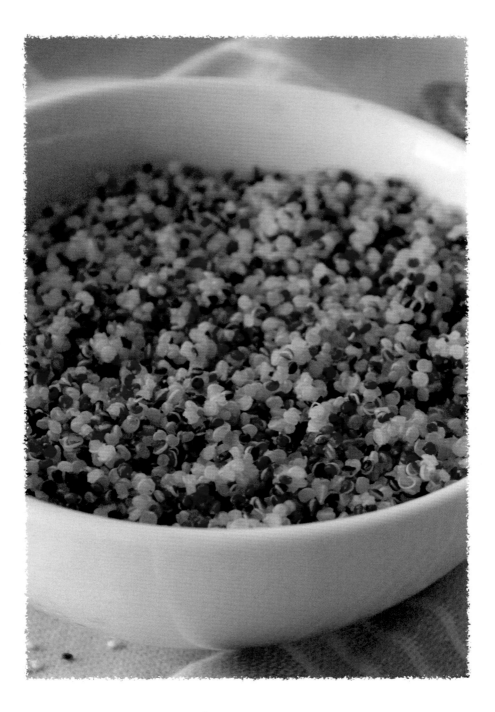

Brown Rice

(Makes 1 cup)

Ingredients:

- ¾ cup Basmati brown rice
- ½ lemon or 1 lime
- 1 tbsp butter
- 2 ½ cup chicken broth or water
- 1 tsp dried thyme
- Sea salt and pepper, to taste

How?

1. Soak rice overnight in filtered water with juice of ½ lemon or 1 lime.
2. Drain water.
3. Melt butter in a pot over medium heat.
4. Add rice and sauté for about 5 minutes. Stir constantly.
5. Add water or broth, cover and cook over medium heat for 30 minutes or until broth has reduced.
6. Turn off heat and season with sea salt and basil.

Tip: I like using Basmati or long-grain brown rice, they are a little less starchy than short-grain brown rice. For the most part I do my best to minimize my intake of grains. But we are all uniquely made and our bodies have different needs. Some of us work better with a higher intake of protein and fats, and others need more of a balance between proteins and carbs. Listen to your body— it always knows what is best for it.

When eating carbs, is always a good idea to consume them with some type of protein or fat, this way carbs are digested slowly and enter the bloodstream at a moderate rate over a period of several hours. When we eat carbs alone, refined or unrefined, they enter the bloodstream in a rush and the body has to work harder to bring sugar levels back to normal. A constant disruption of this fine-tuned system can lead to adrenal fatigue, eventually causing further complications in our health. To learn more, refer to the Breakdown on Sugars under the Real Food Guide section.

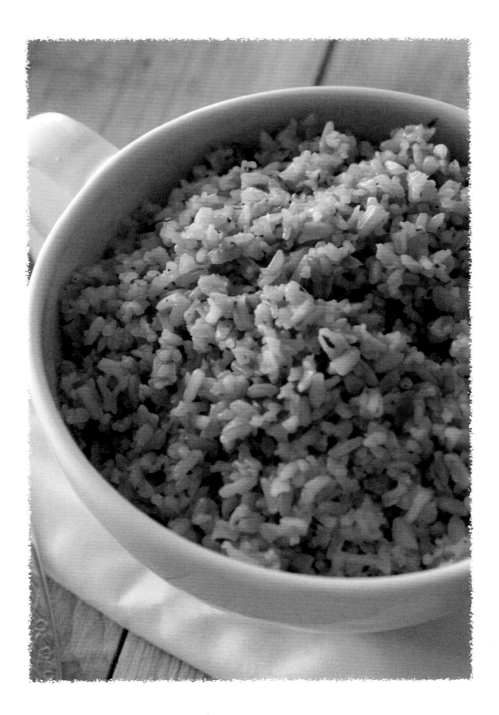

Stuffed Potatoes

(Makes 3-4 people)

Ingredients:

- 4 medium gold potatoes
- 2 tbsp cream cheese
- 1 egg
- 3 tbsp grated parmesan cheese
- 1 tbsp raw milk or coconut milk
- 1 tbsp basil, chopped
- ¼ tsp garlic powder
- Sea salt and ground black pepper, to taste

How?

1. Preheat oven to 350F.
2. Cook potatoes for 15 minutes in boiling water.
3. When potatoes are done allow them to cool enough to be handled.
4. Cut potatoes in half and carefully scoop out the flesh into a bowl.
5. Smash potatoes and combine with cream cheese, egg, 2 tbsp of parmesan and milk.
6. Season with basil, garlic sea salt and pepper.
7. Scoop filling back in each potato and place on a cookie sheet.
8. Sprinkle1 tbsp of parmesan.
9. Bake for 10 minutes and broil for 5 minutes.

Tip: I am sure you can use any other type of potato for this recipe. I prefer gold potatoes because of the size and shape make it easy to scoop out the flesh. Mozzarella or any other cheese works, in case you don't have parmesan handy. Remember, these recipes are to show you that healthy cooking is not complicated, so feel free to replace any ingredients according to your preference.

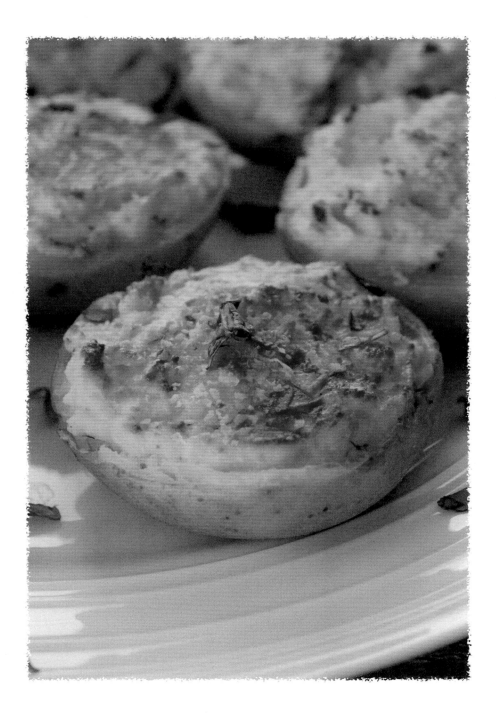

Bacon Brussels Sprouts

(Makes 4 people)

Ingredients:

- 1 lb. brussels sprouts
- 5 bacon strips, chopped
- 1 tsp dried thyme
- 1 tsp garlic powder
- Sea Salt and ground black pepper, to taste

How?

1. Cut brussels sprouts in half.
2. In a pan over medium heat cook bacon for 2 minutes.
3. Add brussels and season with garlic and thyme. Cover and cook for 10 minutes on low heat. Stir constantly to prevent bacon from burning.
4. Season with sea salt and pepper.

Tip: If you are not a pig eater, then bacon can be replaced with turkey bacon.

I love preparing this side for dinner parties because it is so easy to make and goes well with beef, chicken, fish or any other entree.

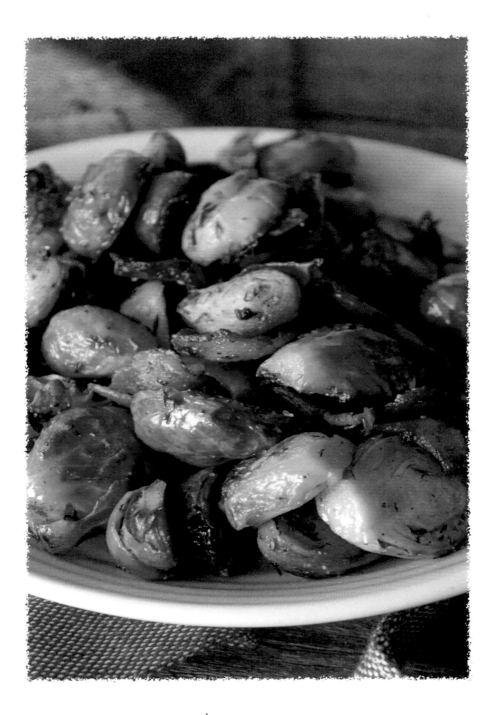

Quinoa Patties

(Makes 5 patties)

Ingredients:

- 1 cup cooked quinoa (white, red quinoa or mixed)
- 1 egg
- ½ tbsp dried basil to taste
- ½ tsp powdered garlic
- ½ tsp sea salt

How?

1. Preheat the oven to 350°F.
2. Mix all the ingredients in a bowl.
3. Place parchment paper over a baking sheet.
4. Form patties with a spoon. It will yield approximately 5 quinoa patties.
5. Bake 7-10 minutes per side.

Tip: If you are in the process of removing or reducing breads and refined carbs from your diet then you are going to love these patties! For me, they satisfied my carb cravings when I decided to cut real bread out of my diet. They are perfect to make sandwiches. You can spread some avocado, top with sliced turkey, make an egg sandwich, melt some cheese on them or simple spread some butter. They are delicious and I'm sure you are going to enjoy them.

You can prepare a batch of quinoa patties and keep them in the fridge for a couple of days or in the freezer for a longer period of time.

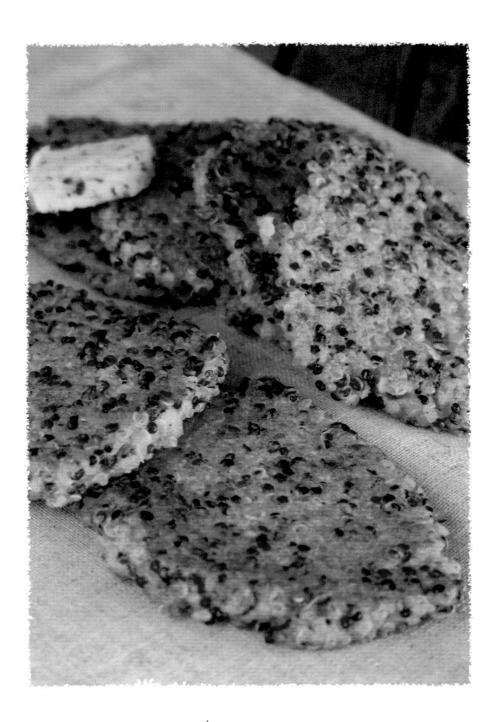

Quinoa Pilaf

(Makes 4)

Ingredients:

- 2 cups cooked quinoa
- 1 tomato, finely chopped
- 8 pitted dates, finely chopped
- 1 pear or red apple, finely chopped
- 2 tbsp fresh cilantro, finely minced
- 5 tbsp fresh basil, finely minced
- 1 handful sliced almonds
- Juice of ½ lemon
- 2 tbsp olive oil
- ¼ tsp garlic powder
- Sea salt and black ground pepper to taste

How?

Mix all ingredients together in a bowl.

Tip: If you want to impress friends and family, this quinoa pilaf is sure to do that. You can definitely prepare it in advance. It stores well in the fridge for 1-2 days; after that the pear is going to start to brown and it won't look too appealing. But I am sure that it won't last that long. This side is guaranteed to satisfy lots of tastebuds!

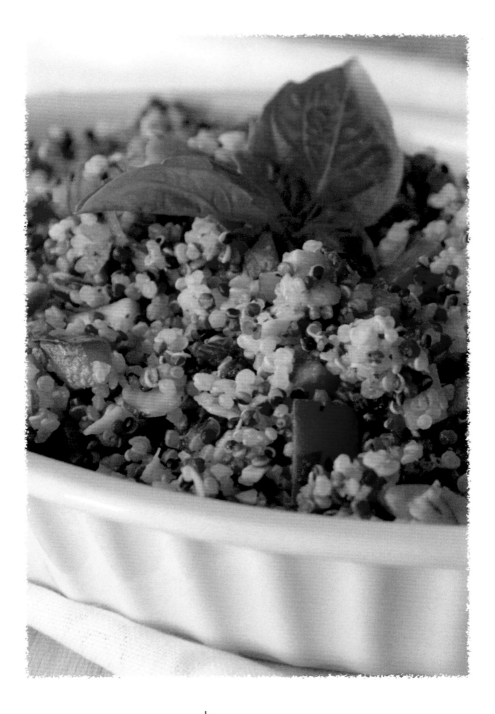

Green Bean Sauté

(Serves 4)

Ingredients:
- 1 tbsp butter
- 1 lb. fresh green beans
- 10 crimini or white mushrooms, sliced
- Sea salt and ground black pepper, to taste
- 4 tsp garlic powder
- 5 fresh basil leaves, finely chopped
- 4 tbsp grated parmesan or shredded mozzarella

How?

1. Melt butter in a pan over medium heat.
2. Add green beans, cover, and sauté for about 5 minutes or until soft, but still crunchy.
3. Add mushrooms and cook until for 3 minutes.
4. Season with garlic powder, sea salt and pepper.
5. Turn off heat.
6. Add basil and cheese.

Tip: Any kind of cheese works well in this recipe. For the majority of the recipes in this book that call for cheese, I use parmesan and mozzarella because I feel they pair well with all different spices and flavors, but definitely feel free to substitute these cheeses for any other type you like.

It is all about having fun. If you ever feel that any of the recipes can be improved by substituting some of the ingredients, then go for it! Be adventurous and fearless in your kitchen.

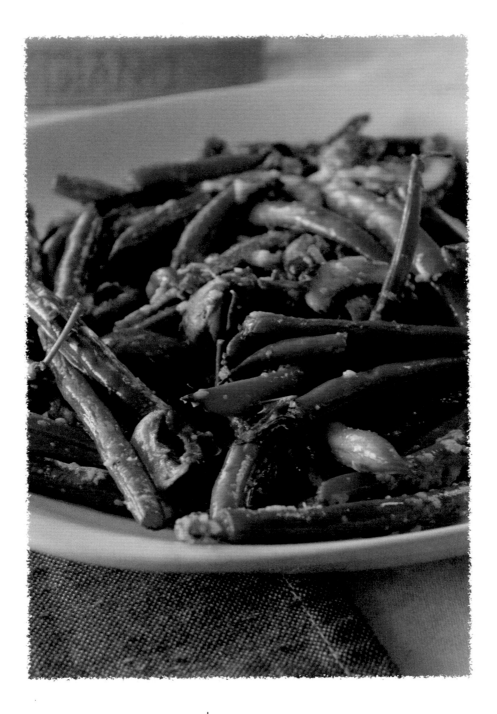

Cauliflower Tortillas

(Makes 10 small tortillas)

Ingredients:

- 1 small cauliflower head
- 3 eggs
- ¼ tsp. garlic powder
- ¼ dried basil
- ¼ tsp. sea salt
- ¼ ground black pepper

How?

1. Preheat oven to 350°F.
2. Cut cauliflower florets and discard stems.
3. Place in food processor and grind cauliflower florets until they reach a rice–like consistency. It should yield 2 cups.
4. Place cauliflower in bowl and using a fork mix with eggs, garlic powder, basil, sea salt, and pepper.
5. Lay parchment paper on baking sheet and with a spoon start forming cauliflower tortillas. It should yield about 10 tortillas.
6. Place baking sheet on the middle rack of the oven. Bake for about 7 minutes each side.

Tip: Once tortillas are done, heat a skillet over medium heat and brown tortillas both sides (less than 30 seconds per side).

You can definitely try to make them bigger than what is suggested in this recipe. The reason I prefer to make them small is because they tend to break easily.

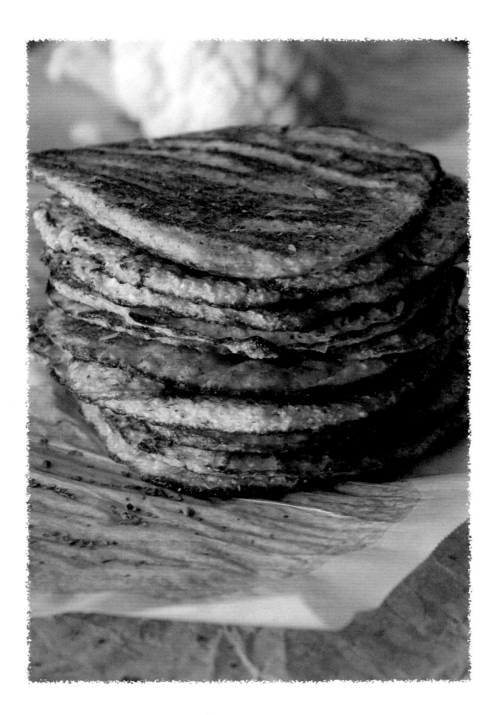

Sweet Potato Wedges
(Makes 2-3)

Ingredients:

- 2 medium-sized sweet potato, peeled
- 1 tbsp coconut oil, melted
- ⅓ tsp powder garlic
- ⅓ tsp dried basil
- Sea Salt and black pepper to taste

How?

1. Preheat oven to 350°F.
2. Cut sweet potatoes into ¼" inch sticks and place in a large bowl.
3. Mix sweet potato with melted coconut oil and spices.
4. Lay sticks on a baking sheet covered with parchment paper.
5. Bake for 15 minutes.

Tip: These sweet potatoes go great with a side of sweet onion dip (Recipe in Dressings section) and are a perfect accompaniment for baked chicken drumsticks (Recipe in Chicken section).

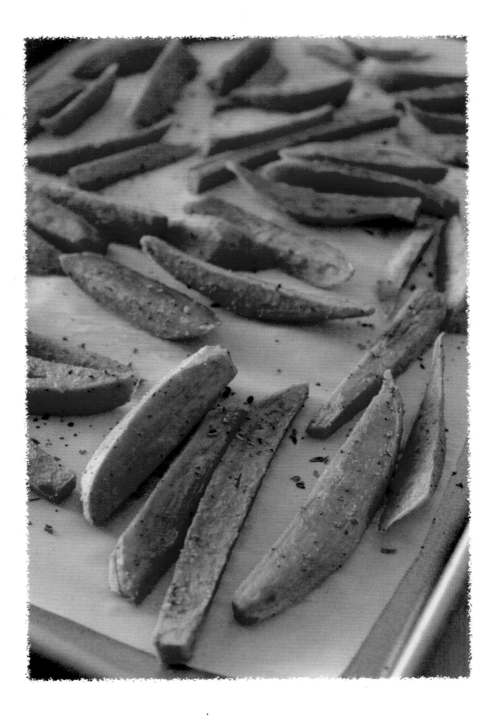

Tomato Avocado Salad

(Makes 2)

Ingredients:
- 1 avocado
- 1 Roma tomato
- Sea salt and ground black pepper, to taste
- 1 tsp olive oil
- 1 tsp lemon juice

How?

1. Chop tomato and avocado (not too small)
2. Season with sea salt and pepper.
3. Drizzle with olive oil and lemon juice.

Tip: This salad goes well on a quinoa patty, cauliflower tortilla or as a side for any chicken and fish dishes.

I borrowed and simplified this recipe from my grandma Maria, who was an extraordinary cook. She was definitely a natural in the kitchen; no matter what she made, it was guaranteed to be a crowdpleaser. I wish I had paid more attention to her cooking methods when I was younger. It is true that sometimes we take for granted what we have in the present. Enjoy the now, your family, your friends, your life, and this recipe!

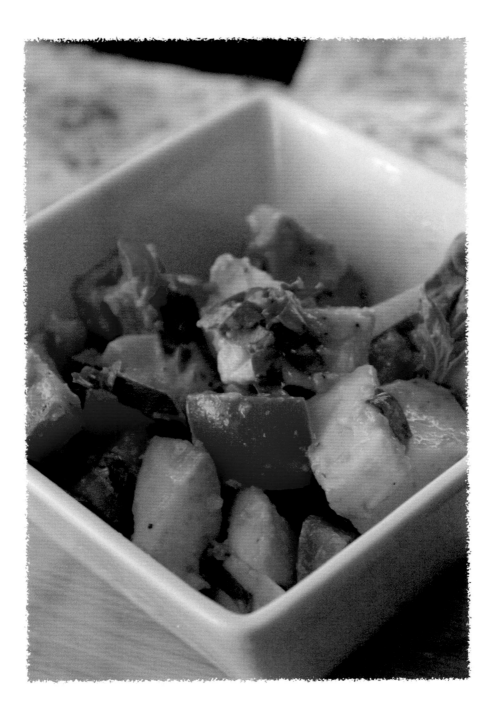

Dressings

Homemade Mayonnaise

Basic Dressing

Kombucha Dressing

Sweet Onion Dip

Homemade Mayonnaise

(Makes ¾ cup)

Ingredients:
- 1 whole egg at room temperature
- 1 egg yolk
- Juice of ½ lemon
- ½ tsp sea salt
- ½ tsp ground black pepper
- ¾ cup avocado oil

How?

1. Place all ingredients in food processor, except the avocado oil.
2. Pulse for about 30 seconds and slowly add avocado oil.
3. Feel free to adjust amounts to your taste preference.

Tip: If you like to give this recipe a twist, add 4-5 fresh basil leaves.

You can definitely use olive oil instead of avocado oil, just make sure to use regular olive oil because extra virgin is a little too strong for my taste.

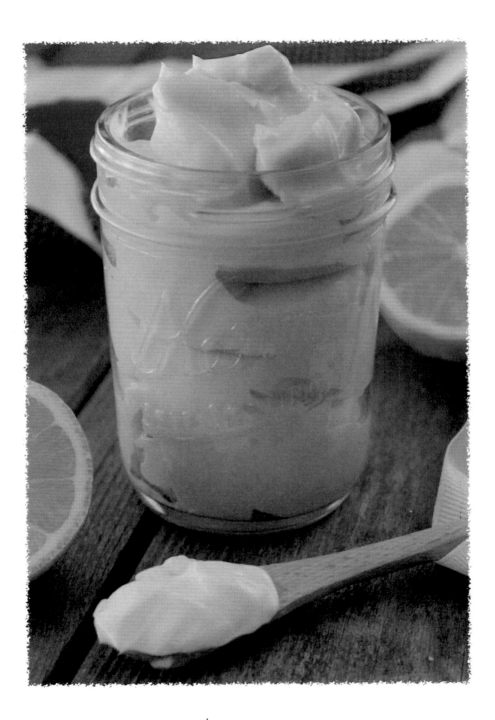

Basic Dressing

(Makes 1 cup)

Ingredients:

- ¾ cup olive oil
- ¼ cup lemon juice
- ½ tsp honey or maple syrup
- ½ tsp sea salt
- ½ tsp cumin
- ½ tsp black pepper
- 1 tsp dried basil
- 1 tsp powdered garlic

How?

Whisk all ingredients together vigorously with a fork. Or pour ingredients in a bottle with lid on and shake content until all ingredients are well mixed.

Tip: When buying olive oil make sure it comes in a dark glass bottle because most unsaturated fats become rancid when exposed to light and high temperatures. Rancid oils are characterized by free radicals, which are extremely reactive. Free radicals are considered "marauders" in the body because they attack cell membranes and red blood cells. They cause wrinkles in the skin, premature aging, set the stage for tumors, and initiate the build up of plaque.

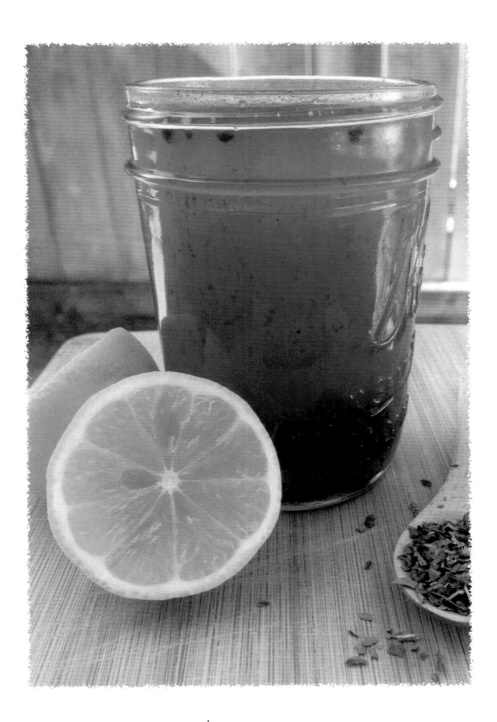

Kombucha Dressing

(Makes 1 cup)

Ingredients:

- ¼ cup kombucha
- ¾ cup olive oil
- 3 tbsp coconut aminos
- ¼ tsp cumin
- ½ tsp oregano
- ¼ tsp sea salt
- ¼ tsp black ground pepper

How?

Whisk all ingredients together with a fork or whisk until it acquires a creamy texture. Pour dressing in a bottle and store it in the refrigerator for several days.

Tip: I cannot emphasize enough the importance of consuming healthy fats. Fats are the building blocks for cell membranes and hormones. Poor quality of cell membrane can lead to body's dysfunctions and other symptoms that make the body more vulnerable to diseases.

The wrong types of fats (saturated fats and monounsaturated) have been vilified for so many decades and refined, commercialized and rancid vegetable oils have been promoted as the "healthy" option for far too long. These types of low quality vegetable oils, (soybean, safflower, cottonseed, canola oil and such) tend to have too much omega 6. High amounts of omega 6 in the diet can cause high tendency to form blood clots, inflammation, high blood pressure, irritation of digestive tract, weak immune function, sterility, cell proliferation, cancer and weight gain. More information can be found in Eat Fat, Be Thin under the Real Food Guide section. If what your reading in these paragraphs is a shocking surprise, I encourage you to read "Eat Fat, Lose Fat" by Mary Enig; I am positive it will change the way you see fats.

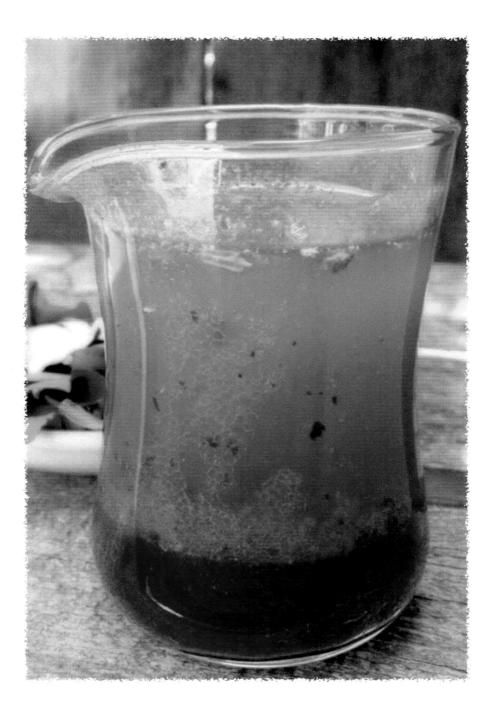

Sweet Onion Dip

(Makes 1 cup)

Ingredients:

- 2 tbsp butter
- 1 medium sweet onion, thinly sliced
- 2 garlic cloves, finely chopped
- 1 tsp yellow mustard
- ½ tbsp apple cider vinegar
- 2 tbsp raw honey
- ½ tsp garlic powder
- Sea salt, to taste
- 1 cup homemade mayonnaise

How?

1. Melt butter in a frying pan or skillet.
2. Add onions and sauté at a medium temperature for about 5 minutes or until they start to brown. Make sure you stir constantly to prevent the onions from burning.
3. Add garlic and cook for about 3 minutes.
4. Place onions and garlic in a food processor and add the rest of the ingredients except mayonnaise, then pulse to blend all ingredients thoroughly.
5. Pour mixture in a bowl and mix with mayonnaise.

Tip: To close this section I would like to explain a little why I am such a big fan of butter, in particular grass-fed. Fat-soluble vitamins A, D, K and E are found in butter in a form that are more easily absorbed and utilized. These vitamins are exceptionally important because they allow our bodies to use the vitamins we consume, either through food or supplements. Vitamin A and D are essential for growth, healthy bones, nervous system, development of brain and normal sexual development. Vitamin A, D, K and E protect us from calcification of joints - arthritis, calcification of arteries, cataracts and calcification of pineal gland, which is responsible for production of melatonin (hormone that plays an important role in the regulation of sleep cycles). In the Real Food Guide you will find more information about the importance and benefits of saturated fats and brief explanation about cholesterol.

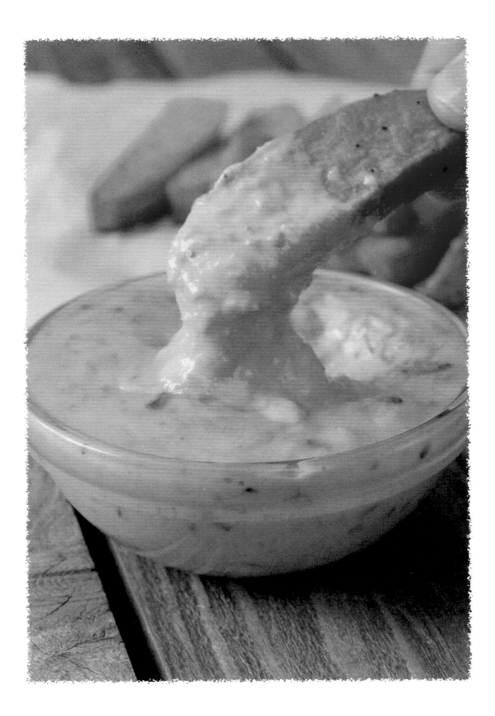

Something Sweet

Flourless Carrot Cake

Raspberry Cashew Pie

Almond Coconut Balls

Coconut Whipped Cream

Nutty Chocolate Bark

Double-Layer Sweet Potato Cake

A dessert, especially one made with healthy ingredients, is not going to kill you once in a while. Even though you may be tempted to indulge in an occasional sweet at a restaurant, you are better off making it at home. That way, you know exactly what is in it and can use alternative sweeteners instead of refined white sugar. Make sure to always control your sugar intake even if it comes from natural sources. The key to life is balance, and many (including me) cannot strike a balance without dessert.

Flourless Carrot Cake

Ingredients:

- ¾ cup cup dried pinto beans
- 2 cups water
- 1 cup raisins
- 1 cup coconut palm sugar
- ¾ cup coconut oil, melted
- 2 eggs
- 1 tsp baking soda
- 1 tsp ground cinnamon
- ½ tsp sea salt
- 1 cup carrots, peeled and shredded (approx. 2 large carrots)

Cinnamon glaze ingredients:

- 5 tbsp coconut milk
- ½ tsp ground cinnamon
- ½ cup coconut sugar
- Soak ¾ dried pinto beans, it will yield to 1½ cup after soaked overnight.

How?

1. Soak pinto beans in warm water with some lemon juice overnight. Rinse and drain. Place pinto beans and water in a pot. Let boil, skim, and cover. Lower temperature to medium-low heat and simmer for about half an hour. Turn off heat and cool. Discard any leftover water.
2. Preheat oven to 350°F.
3. Place raisins in a bowl and cover with hot water.
4. Place a sheet of parchment paper on the bottom of a 9-inch round baking pan and grease the sides with coconut oil.
5. In a food processor, mix pinto beans, coconut sugar, coconut oil, and eggs. Process until a smooth batter has formed.
6. Then add baking soda, cinnamon and sea salt and mix well.
7. Drain raisins and add to the batter along with the carrots.
8. Process until it is evenly distributed.
9. Pour mix into the prepared baking pan and bake for about 45 to 55 minutes or until able to insert a fork and it comes out clean. Remove from oven and let cool. Loosen the sides with a knife and quickly flip the cake onto a platter. Discard parchment paper.

Cinnamon glaze:

1. Heat coconut milk, cinnamon, and coconut sugar over low heat until well combined.
2. Simmer for about 3 minutes.
3. Cover carrot cake with glaze.
4. Serve immediately or place in the refrigerator for 30 minutes. It is also delicious when is cold.

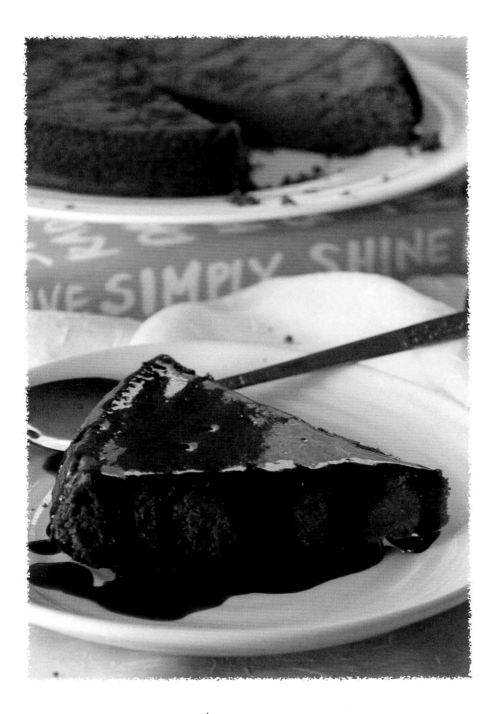

Raspberry Cashew Pie

ingredients:

Crust
- 2 cups cashews, soaked
- 10 black figs
- 1 tsp cocoa powder

Filling:
- 2 cups cashews, soaked
- ¼ cup lemon juice
- ½ cup maple syrup
- ¾ cup unrefined coconut oil, melted
- ½ cup frozen raspberries

How?

1. Soak nuts overnight in warm water with some lemon juice.
2. Drain and discard water.
3. Place all other crust ingredients in food processor and mix well until a dough-like consistency has formed.
4. Line a sheet of parchment paper or aluminum foil in a 9-inch round baking pan.
5. Now, press the nuts and figs mixture down into the pan to form the crust.
6. Place all the filling ingredients in the food processor and blend until a creamy consistency has been reached.
7. Pour the mixture into the pan and freeze for about an hour.

Tip: If you are not a fan of raspberries, then feel free to substitute with any other fruit of your choice. I have made this pie using mangos and the taste is amazing.

One more thing: figs can be replaced with dates, the only difference is that it will be little sweeter.

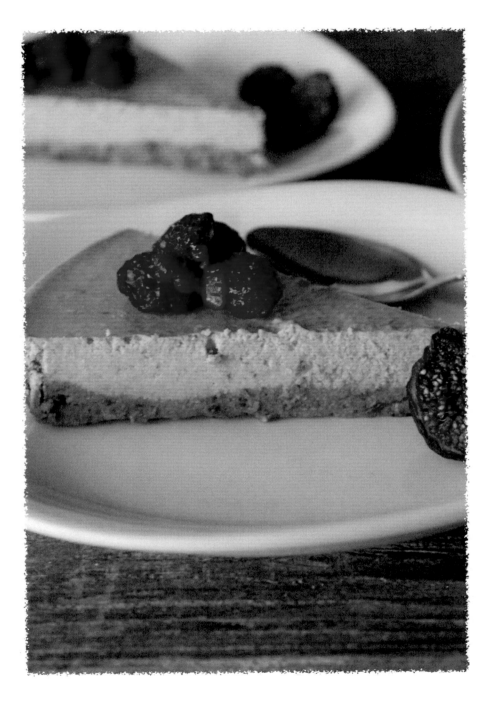

Almond Coconut Balls

(Makes 10 small balls)

. . . .

Ingredients:

- 1½ cup unsweetened shredded coconut
- ½ cup shaved almonds
- 4 tbsp almond butter

- 2 tsp vanilla extract
- 1½ tbsp maple syrup
- 2 tsp coconut oil, melted.
- Pinch of sea salt

. . . .

How?

1. Place all ingredients in food processor.
2. Pulse until all ingredients until they are completely blended.
3. Grab small portions of the dough and roll into 10 balls.
4. Place on a plate and freeze for about 10 minutes.

Tip: Having healthy snack available at home makes it easier to maintain a healthy diet. When your body asks for food, it seems as if the brain blocks and the only thing working are the physical cravings, so for that reason I like to have healthy snacks ready in the fridge. These little balls are so easy to make and are free of refined sugars and refined oils. Of course, there are exceptions to the rule, there are brands that do care about the ingredients they use.

It is always a good idea to keep consumption of sugars and carbs low because even though they are sources of quick energy, the excess will be stored in the body as fat. You can read all the complications that sugars and carbs, especially refined, cause to the body, just flip back to the Real Food Guide section.

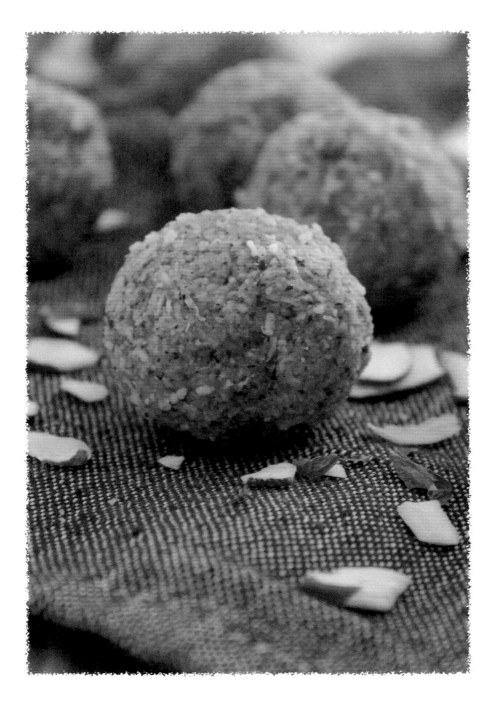

Coconut Whipped Cream

(Makes 1 cup)

Ingredients:
- 1 can full-fat coconut cream, chilled
- 3-4 tsp honey, coconut syrup or maple syrup
- ½ tsp vanilla extract

How?

1. Chill a can of coconut cream in the refrigerator overnight.
2. Remove cream from can and place in a bowl. Do not include liquid.
3. Fold in coconut syrup and vanilla extract with a spatula.

Tip: If the cream is too hard, use a hand mixer to blend all ingredients.

Don't you love having healthy alternative for all those foods that thrill the tastebuds? I can eat this whipped cream with a couple of strawberries or mixed with berries. This creamy concoction will bring any dessert to the next level!

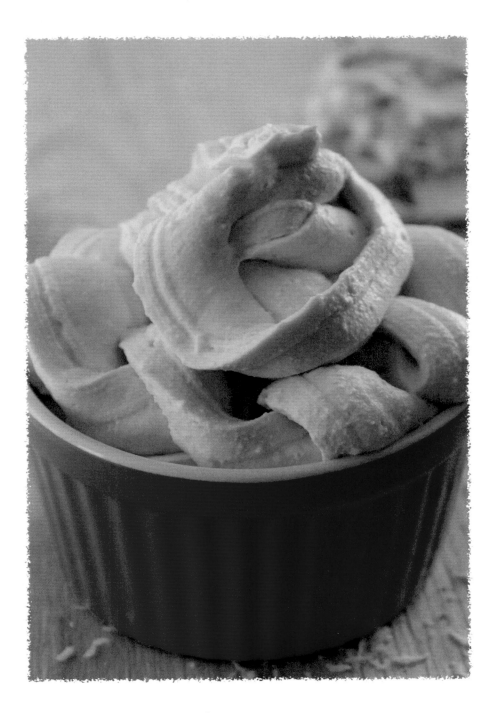

Nutty Chocolate Bark

Ingredients:
- ¾ cup coconut oil, melted
- 3 tbsp raw cacao powder
- 2 tsp maple syrup or honey
- ⅓ cup sliced almonds
- ⅓ cup pecan pieces

How?

1. Mix melted coconut oil and cacao powder.
2. Add maple syrup and continue mixing.
3. Cover an 8-inch skillet with aluminum foil.
4. Place almonds and pecans on skillet and distribute evenly to cover the surface.
5. Pour in chocolate mixture.
6. Lift and swirl the skillet to cover nuts.
7. Place in freezer for 10 minutes

Tip: Feel free to adjust maple syrup and cacao powder amounts. I like very dark chocolate, so if you are more of a milk-chocolate person, then try with 1 or 2 tbsp of cacao powder.

I never feel guilty eating this chocolate because the primary ingredient is coconut oil. Coconut oil has so many benefits, my favorite is that it has anti-fungal, anti-bacterial and anti-viral properties. It contains lauric acid, which protects the gut from external pathogens. I use coconut oil for everything: for cooking, as my daily morning drink, make-up remover, skin lotion, as shaving cream and I even use it on my hair. Coconut oil should definitely be in everyone's pantry. To learn more on how I use coconut oil refer to Supplements for Health section and Daily Facial and Body Care section.

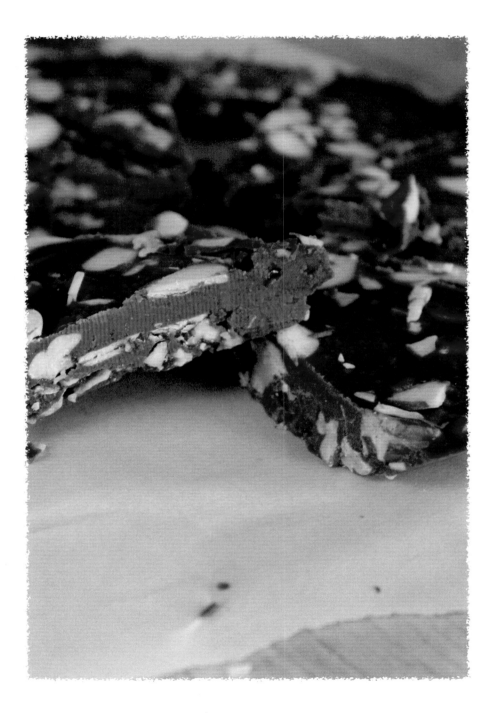

Double Layer Sweet Potato Cake

Ingredients:

- 2 medium-sized sweet potatoes (or 2 cups)
- 4 tbsp maple syrup
- ½ cup coconut flour
- 4 tbsp coconut oil
- 6 eggs
- 2 tsp vanilla extract
- 2 tbsp cacao powder

How?

1. Preheat oven to 350°F.
2. Line a sheet of parchment paper on a 9" round baking pan and grease sides with coconut oil. Set aside.
3. In a pot, boil water and add sweet potato. Cook for about 15 minutes or until tender.
4. Allow sweet potatoes too cool and then peel skins off.
5. Mash sweet potatoes.
6. In a food processor place 1 cup of mashed sweet potato, 2 tbsp maple syrup, ¼ cup coconut flour, 3 eggs, 1 tsp vanilla extract, and 2 tbsp coconut oil. Pulse until all ingredients are well combined.
7. Pour mixture in baking pan.
8. Repeat step 5 and include cacao powder.
9. Pour chocolate mixture as a second layer. Using a spatula spread the mixture to cover the surface.
10. Place in oven and bake for 45 minutes.
11. Allow it to cool at room temperature then chill in the refrigerator.
12. Top with coconut whipped cream.

Tip: Add coconut whipped cream to take this dessert to another level. This dessert is definitely a crowd pleaser. It is so delicious that it is hard to believe that it is only made of sweet potatoes. You'll have your family and friends wanting more.

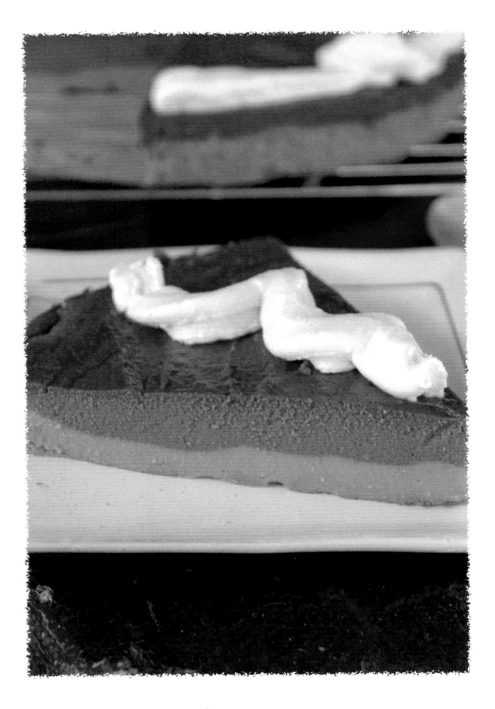

Supplements for health

These suggestions are based on the recommendations I have been given and what has worked for me. It is always a good idea to consult with a health professional to make sure these supplements will also be beneficial for you. Remember, we are all uniquely made and our bodies have different needs.

Magnesium

It is difficult to obtain enough magnesium from real food because farm soil is largely depleted from this essential mineral. For this reason, I supplement with magnesium daily to ensure that I am getting enough. Every single cell in the body requires magnesium in order to function properly. It helps keep our bones and teeth strong, balances our hormones, and maintains a healthy nervous and cardiovascular system. Magnesium also relaxes the body and muscles, which promotes better sleep. It is also essential for heart and brain health.

Stress consumes large amounts of magnesium and if we do not replenish our bodies' supplies, we could experience the many effects of magnesium deficiency. Because it is so difficult to obtain enough magnesium from food, deficiencies are very common; symptoms include asthma, arthritis, constipation, dental cavities, depression, type I and II diabetes, heart disease, insomnia, migraines, fatigue, muscle cramping, and thyroid disorders (just to name a few).

Great sources of this essential element are nuts, avocados, unrefined sea salt, sprouted grains, and legumes. However, as I mentioned, it is difficult to get enough magnesium from food. There are many types of magnesium supplements, but magnesium malate or citrate are easier for the body to absorb. The brand I have been using for more than five years is Magnesium Malate-Chelate from Designs for Health.

Cod Liver Oil

If you have heard of fish oil, fermented cod liver oil is its overachieving cousin. Fermentation protects the naturally occurring nutrients in the cod liver oil, including omega-3 fatty acids and vitamins A and D. The fermentation process also makes the nutrients in foods and supplements easier for our bodies to digest and absorb. Unlike fermented cod liver oil, fish oil is not processed in this way, meaning many of its nutrients are damaged or lost.

Furthermore, recent studies have shown that there is no long-term benefit of taking fish oil and that it can, in fact, be harmful to your health. While the purpose of taking fish oil is to consume fatty acids EPA and DHA in large doses (which is proving to be potentially unsafe), the point of taking fermented cod liver oil is to increase your consumption of fat-soluble vitamins A, D, K2, and E in balanced ratios. These essential nutrients can be difficult to obtain in modern diets, as most of us do not consume large quantities of organ meat, which is one of the few major sources of these vitamins. Therefore, it is especially helpful to supplement on a daily basis with fermented cod liver oil. Here is a list of benefits of this amazing superfood (from Dr. Ron's Ultra-Pure website):

- Auto-immune booster
- Transports calcium to joints and bones
- Best source on earth of vitamins A and D in a perfect ratio
- Enhances and maintains brain function – yes! It helps stop degeneration!
- Regulates blood pressure and cholesterol naturally
- Great source of omega-3
- Eases pain and inflammation in the body – joint, pain, arthritis
- Enhances ability to sleep through the night
- Helps fight depression
- It is in rich in enzymes, nutrients, vitamin K & E, Coenzyme Q10 and other important biological molecules.

Probiotics

Lacto-fermented foods and raw dairy, in articular raw kefir, are nature's best sources of probiotics. Maintaining a healthy gut is extremely important for overall health, and it is difficult (if not impossible) to have a healthy gut without consuming probiotic foods. You can read about the benefits of probiotic foods in the Healing Foods section.

If you don't consume many fermented foods or raw dairy, it may be a good idea to add probiotics supplements to your routine. I have tried different brands and the ones that have worked better for me are the ones that have a variety of bacterial strains and additive free. However, because the bacterial strands in probiotics vary so greatly and serve different purposes, it may be wise to seek the help of a holistic or other medical practitioner, who will be able to recommend the best probiotic for you based on your diet, lifestyle, and current health condition.

Coconut oil

Coconut oil is one of my favorite multi-purpose supplements. Its uses are literally endless and I use it and consume it on a daily basis. Every morning, I dilute a spoonful of coconut oil in a warm cup of water and drink it on an empty stomach. This activates the digestive system and boosts the immune system. Coconut oil has antibacterial and antiviral properties and is also a good source of healthy fat, so you stay satisfied and energetic throughout your morning. Coconut oil water is also used by people who are looking to lose weight. In this case, drink a cup of coconut oil water half an hour before meals. It takes few tries to get use to coconut oil water, so if the taste bothers you then start with a teaspoon.

Coconut oil is also a great and safe cooking oil because of its high smoke point. It is a perfect butter replacement in baking and also is the best moisturizer, acne treatment, and hair conditioner. Many people also oil pull with coconut oil. All you have to do is put a tablespoon of coconut oil in your mouth and swish it around for 15 minutes, then spit it out and brush your teeth. The coconut oil removes the harmful bacteria in your mouth and is also a great remedy for bad breath. The uses for coconut oil are truly endless— you will find countless others online.

Adrenal Support

Stress is one of the main reasons for illness. Life happens and difficult situations arise unexpectedly. Also, we are often stressed on a daily basis without even realizing it. Stress wreaks havoc on our adrenal glands, which control many of our bodily functions. Therefore, it is important to protect them.

Whenever I am working long hours, not able to get enough rest, or I am experiencing emotional stress, I like to help my body with adrenal support supplements. The supplement that works well for me is Adrenal Rebuilder by Doctor Wilson's.

*Just a quick note:

The supplements I consume are free of gluten, yeast, soy, artificial coloring, flavoring and preservatives. The reason I am mentioning some of the brands it is not for marketing purposes, but because I have tried them for several years, have experienced their benefits, and therefore feel confident recommending them.

High quality supplements can tend to cost more than synthetic supplements. I would suggest you to do your own research and do not feel limited to these brands. Visit your health food stores and browse the supplement aisles or poke around online. One of the websites I use to order some of the supplements mentioned is Natural Healthy Concepts.

Daily Facial & Body Care

Body Care Products

Your skin is your body's largest organ. Anything that you put on it will be absorbed into your bloodstream. Whenever I shop for toiletries, I look for the following characteristics:

- Paraben free
- Won't clog pores or non-comedogenic
- Sulfate free
- No perfume
- Organic

There are a lot of great brands for face and body care. You can purchase them at health stores or online. The Environmental Working Group, a nonprofit consumer advocacy organization, has a cosmetics database that rates products for safety. This is a great way to see exactly what is in your products and whether or not they are safe. If you find that your products are not as safe as you would hope, it is a great way to find new products and support brands that protect their customers' health. Visit www.ewg.org/skindeep

Organic makeup

Everyone's makeup preferences and routines are different. I try to keep things simple; a little foundation and blush is enough for me. If you use foundation, always try to stick with a product that won't clog pores (non-comedogenic), and organic is best. I use Afterglow makeup, which applies smoothly and feels so light on the skin. If you're in the process of healing your skin, try to go without makeup while you are at home in order to let it breathe as much as possible. It will thank you for giving it a break.

Coconut oil night cream/make-up remover

I am a coconut oil lover! I eat it, cook with it, put it on my skin, my hair, and use it as a makeup remover. It is simply amazing! Besides its many health benefits, coconut oil is my beauty partner. I use it as an eye makeup remover. It does not burn my eyes and smoothly removes mascara, eyeliner, and eyeshadow. A little bit goes a long way, so you really don't need much.

I also use it as a night facial cream. First, wash your face and let your skin dry for about five minutes. Rub a pea-sized amount of coconut oil between your hands and gently massage your face. Your skin will absorb it really fast.

Coconut oil's antibacterial and antifungal properties will help your skin heal faster. If you have a pimple, it will help it mature faster, but don't pop it, just continue with using coconut oil as your night cream and it will go away on its own. It also helps with scars from blemishes. You just have to be consistent and patient. Feel free to put it all over your body too; it makes a wonderful moisturizer.

Coconut Facial Wash

I have tried several facial washes that are organic, paraben-free, and made with pure ingredients. They all work great, but frankly, coconut oil has been my favorite so far. One time I ran out of my facial wash and remembered watching a video online of a girl using coconut oil to wash her face, so I gave it a try and fell in love with this method! All you need is the following:

- ½ tsp coconut oil
- 1 small towel
- Bowl of warm water

Simply wet your face and rub coconut oil on for about a minute. Wet towel in warm water, wring it out, and place on your face for 15 seconds. Softly clean coconut oil off and repeat one more time. If you do it in the morning, feel free to use your regular moisturizer afterwards and if done at night you can rub a little coconut oil on your face as your night cream.

Kombucha mask

I used these recipes from Kombucha Kamp. Kombucha masks will make your skin feel smooth and look sun-kissed. If you have any blemishes it will help them mature faster, and because it is a living organism, the SCOBY will help regenerate skin cells.

Option 1:

1 SCOBY

Wash your face. Please a SCOBY on your face. Don't worry; it won't eat your brains out. Leave it on for about 15-30 minutes while you relax. Remove SCOBY and rinse your face.

Assign a separate glass container to store your facial SCOBY in. Please don't use it to make kombucha!

Option 2:

1 SCOBY

1 egg

In a food processor place all ingredients and blend. It should be a chunky paste. Place paste on a clean face and let it dry for about 15 minutes. Your face might be a little red afterwards (like a sunburn), but it doesn't take long to fade away.

*Just a quick note:

If you are suffering from acne like I was or experiencing any other skin problems, please always keep in mind that what is truly going to heal your condition are the changes in your nutrition. Your inner health is reflected on your skin. These are simply tips to help you through the healing process, but problematic skin will most likely persist until your gut health improves through nutrition and healthy lifestyle.

Proven one more time— nature works!

To prove what I just mentioned on the quick note above, let me tell you briefly about a recent experience.

I went on a 20-day trip to Europe. It was a lot of fun, but also included eating out every day, trying all types of food and alcohol, and sleeping little— all things that my body was not used to at all. When I came back, I began to notice that I was breaking out again around my chin area, so without thinking twice, I put myself back on track.

I began my mornings with a cup of warm coconut water with a tablespoon of coconut oil, and then started juicing every morning. I went back to consuming kefir for breakfast and made some chicken bone stock and kombucha, which I consumed with every meal. I missed them so much! I also greatly increased my water intake.

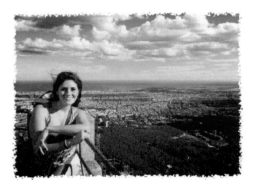

I went back to my yoga class and became more active again. And of course went back to cooking my own meals. Lastly, but not least, I let my body rest its 8 hours and tried my best to go to sleep before 11:00 pm.

On the outside, I was using kombucha masks. It is really amazing how it works. It makes any breakouts mature much faster.

With persistence and continuity, again my body began to heal. After a couple of days, my skin began to look much better and after a week, everything was pretty much gone.

There is absolutely no doubt that your body will heal on its own by treating yourself right and eating healthy. Try it! And give nature a chance!

Open your mind:

When I started this nutritional journey, I thought I would only see changes in my physical health. I was totally unaware that the changes were going to be much deeper. Once I started respecting myself and treating my body as the greatest gift I had, I began noticing that I was not only craving healthy food, but also that my mind was craving positivism, peace, relaxation, focus, inspiration, and connection.

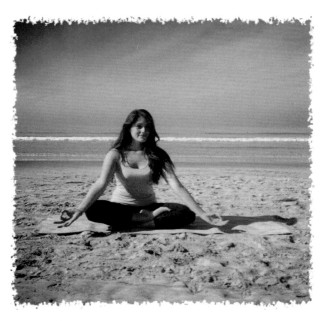

I began attending yoga and meditation classes. At first I took it as an extra activity that I could add to my exercise routine, but now I understand that by feeding my mind with goodness, I was also allowing my body to heal.

I started to understand that mind and body are one; it is too difficult to achieve health with negativity and stress. You can be eating the healthiest diet in the world, but if your mind is congested with bad thoughts, then it will start preventing your body from working the way it is meant to and you will get frustrated because you won't see the results that you are so impatiently waiting to witness.

I began surrounding myself with people who supported me, walking away from drama, and learning to put myself first. And no! It is not selfish to consider yourself as the most important person in your world because you must be balanced and happy before you try to positively influence someone else's life. After all, we are only able to give what we have.

I am aware this is a cooking and health book, but I felt the need to finish these last pages by telling you that you are not only what you eat, but also what you think. Allow yourself to relax and drop expectations, anger, resentfulness and all of those bad feelings that simply feed your ego and hurt your mind.

Here is a list of books that I have read and have taught me valuable lessons about the beauty of being alive.

- Inspiration by Wayne Dyer
- The Passion Test by Janet Attwood
- Your Erroneous Zones by Wayne Dyer
- Real Miracles by Wayne Dyer
- You'll see it when you believe it by Wayne Dyer

My Sources

Throughout my health journey, I read voraciously and learned so much about the connection between nutrition and health, but our bodies are so complex that there is still so much more to learn.

Reading about nutrition became one of my passions. It is incredible how intelligent and amazing our bodies function. We are so perfect and many times we don't realize the power of healing we have within ourselves and ignore that Mother Nature has given us everything we need to obtain vibrant health.

There are a cornucopia of books written by professionals and people like me, who are sharing their experiences and how they were able to change their lives through diet and lifestyle. Below is a list of the books and websites that I have referred in this book because they have had the greatest impact on me and provided me with revolutionary and invaluable information.

- Eat Fats, Lose Fats by Dr. Mary Enig and Sally Fallon
- Nutrition and Physical Degeneration by Weston A. Price
- Nourishing Traditions by Sally Fallon (This one is my kitchen bible)
- How to Make Kombucha Tea by Hannah Crum
- Perspectives in Nutrition by Wardlaw and Insel
- www.mercola.com
- www.westonpricefoundation.com
- www.nourishedkitchen.com
- www.healthhomehappy.com
- www.nomnompaleo.com
- www.everydaypaleo.com
- www.ewg.org

Thank you for reading these pages and for deciding to take care of your most precious asset - You!

Wish you health, love and peace all the way.

Jen - your creative cook and nutrition lover

Download Naked Flavors app for more recipes

Follow Naked Flavors on Instagram and Facebook

www.nakedflavorsnutrition.com

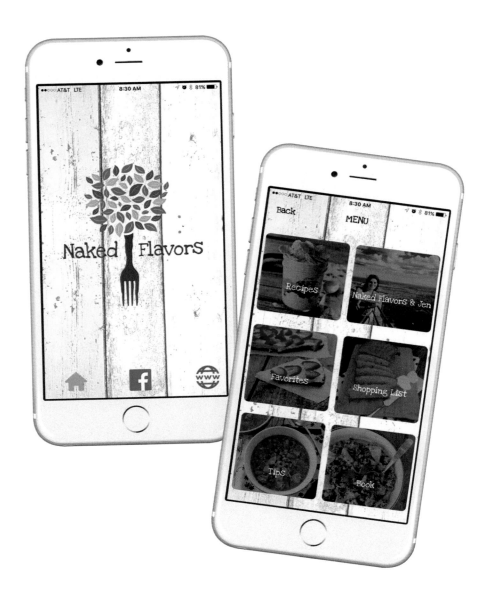

About the Author

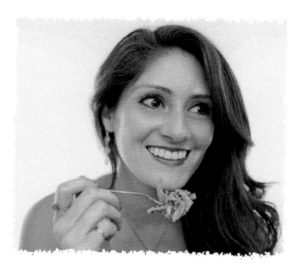

Jeniffer Alburquerque is a certified Nutritional Therapy Practitioner, creator of the healthy recipe app Naked Flavors, fervent advocate of the feel-awesome-everyday movement and a true believer that dancing in the kitchen adds flavor to her healthy concoctions. For many years she struggled with severe acne and several digestive problems that made her feel lousy and purposeless. Her frustration for so many unsuccessful attempts to heal her condition with prescribed and over-the-counter medicine led her making a life changing decision - to give mother nature a chance to cure her. This episode in her life made her discover her great passion for cooking and nutrition. Today Jen spends her time helping those suffering with acne and digestive disorders. She also continues learning about food-body connection in order to create nourishing and tasty recipes with the purpose to inspire others to make the right nutritional choices and understand the power of health.

Visit her at www.nakedflavorsnutrition.com and for more taste bud thrilling recipes download Naked Flavors app.

44899877R10108

Made in the USA
San Bernardino, CA
23 July 2019